ART & AESTHETIC SURGERY

Urs Victor Burki, M.D.

ART & AESTHETIC SURGERY

Benteli

Cover: Urs Victor Burki
Illustrations and drawings: Urs Victor Burki
All the pre- and postoperative photographs represent patients of Urs Victor Burki, M.D.
Translation: David Kevin Whiteley
PrePress: Prolith AG, Schönbühl
Production: Benteli Publishers, Bern

ISBN 3-7165-1352-0
ISBN 978-3-7165-1352-1

Distribution:
Benteli Publishers
Seftigenstrasse 310
CH-3084 Wabern/Bern
Phone ++41 (0)31 960 84 84
Fax ++41 (0)31 961 74 14
info@benteliverlag.ch
www.benteliverlag.ch

Table of contents

Foreword Ivo Pitanguy, M. D. 7

Preface Leo Clodius, M. D. 8

Introduction 11

Leonardo da Vinci – a Rich Source of Inspiration 12

Mona Lisa – her Aesthetic Operation 16

The Quest for Beauty 20

Beauty – in the Eyes of the Philosophers 26

Ideals of Beauty and Facial Proportions 32

- The Classical Greek and Renaissance Ideals of Beauty 32
- Studies on Facial Proportions by Leonardo da Vinci and Albrecht Dürer 35
- My Own Studies of Facial Proportions 44
- Golden Ratio and Fibonacci Sequences Applied to the Face 54
- Symmetry of the Face: a Variable Factor 59
- Observer Distance Determines Facial Proportions 60
- Beauty Resides in the Eye of the Beholder 63

Pioneers of Aesthetic Facial Surgery 64

Aesthetic Facial Surgery 72

- Facial Rejuvenation Surgery 72
- Eyelid Surgery (Blepharoplasty) 76
- Forehead and Eyebrow Lift 78
- Face and Neck Lift 81
- Mini Face Lift (Minimal Incision Face Lift) 84
- Micro Liposuction/Liposculpture 85
- Surface Treatments 86
- Botulinum Toxin 88
- Filling Treatments 90
- Aesthetic Rhinoplasty 92
- Facial Bone Structure Surgery 95
- Aesthetic Otoplasty 97
- Aesthetic Surgery of the Lips 99
- Pre- and Postoperative Considerations 102

The Quest for Perfection in Facial Rejuvenation 110

Face Lift Patients Share Their Experience 128

To all my patients

To all those who believe in innovation

To lovers of beauty

I wish to thank most sincerely all my patients, without whom this book would not have been written.

I would also like to express my gratitude to my mentors, teachers and colleagues who have guided and supported me to evolve constantly in the art of aesthetic surgery of the face:

Aston Sherrell J., M.D., New York, USA
Baker Daniel C., M.D., New York, USA
Baker, Jr., James L., M.D., Winter Park, USA
Baker Thomas J., M.D., Miami, USA
Buff Hans-Ulrich, Prof. Dr. med., Zürich, Switzerland (†)
Connell Bruce F., M.D., Santa Ana, USA
Clodius Leo, PD, Dr. med., Zürich, Switzerland
González-Ulloa Mario, M.D., Prof., Mexico 7, Mexico (†)
Lewis, Jr., John R., M.D., Atlanta, USA (†)
Millard, Jr., Ralph D., M.D., Prof., Miami, USA
Pitanguy Ivo, M.D., Prof., Rio de Janeiro, Brazil
Rees Thomas D., M.D., Prof., New York, USA

Foreword

As plastic surgery has evolved in recent years, the amount of information that the patient should be aware of has increased tremendously. Perhaps the most valuable fact to be transmitted to our patients pertains to the limits of the surgical procedure. The plastic surgeon is sometimes seen as a sculptor of the living tissue, dealing with an individual who rationalizes but has idealizations, someone who is both conscious and unconscious, with a body and soul. Although plastic surgery is a noble branch of general surgery, a proper understanding of the surgeon's limitations is fundamental when assessing aesthetic impairments. A realistic expectation can only be identified once the patient understands that, unlike the sculptor and painter, the plastic surgeon must obey the laws of anatomy and proportion. Harmony and equilibrium are the tools with which the surgeon will attain his results.

In this book, Urs Victor Burki explains to his readers, in clear language, the art and science of plastic surgery, referring to the great artists of the past who enhance our sensitivity; but he also highlights our limits as surgeons.

Ivo Pitanguy

Professor of plastic surgery of the Pontifical Catholic University of Rio de Janeiro (PUC-Rio) and of the Carlos Chagas Institute of Post-Graduate Medical Studies. Member of the Brazilian Society of Plastic Surgery, the National Academy of Medicine and the Brazilian Academy of Letters. Visiting professor I.S.A.P.S., F.A.C.S., F.I.C.S., T.C.B.C.

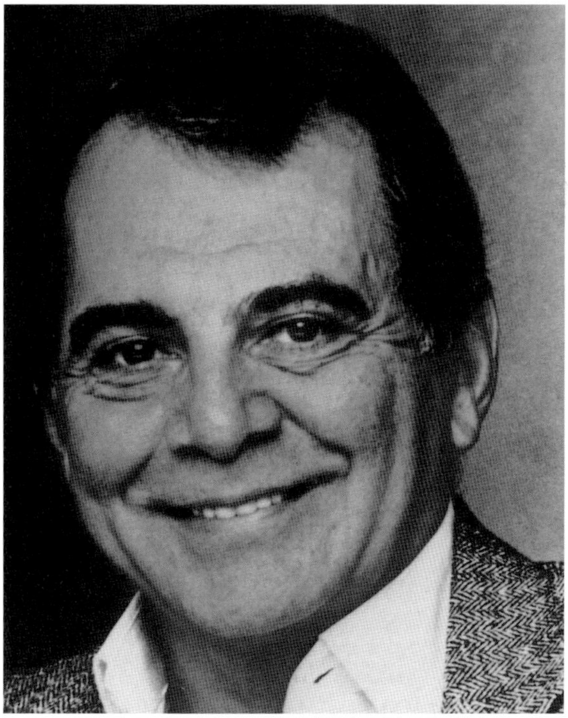

Prof. Ivo Pitanguy, M.D.

Preface

Aesthetic surgery is concerned primarily with what the patient subjectively experiences.
Leo Clodius

Art & Aesthetic Surgery is a book that the public has long been waiting for. It affords the interested reader a comprehensive insight into all the different aspects of facial aesthetic surgery. The patient will be able to find quickly all the relevant information and to consider the fundamental issues. This book can also serve to supplement and complete the information and explanations obtained during the medical consultation.

Some patients mistakenly believe – on account of the often-inadequate information provided in some women's magazines – that a significant facial rejuvenation effect will be achieved simply by removing wrinkles or merely by tightening the skin. This informative and easy-to-read book clearly shows that this assumption is incorrect. Rather, a naturally harmonious appearance is obtained by repositioning certain tissue structures and by judiciously combining the individually appropriate operating techniques.

Urs Victor Burki draws the reader's attention to the specific characteristics of a branch of medicine which does not allow even the slightest error. Only an experienced surgeon pays attention to the minor yet important details that contribute to an excellent result. My former student and co-worker, Urs Victor Burki, achieves astonishing results in facial rejuvenation surgery – as evidenced by the numerous photographs of his patients. He masters the art of attaining a significant and most natural rejuvenation of the face, without altering in the slightest the personal facial features. He thus achieves the supreme objectives of facial aesthetic surgery: naturalness and harmony.

The aspiration to achieve perfection has driven Urs Victor Burki to set important new trends in aesthetic surgery of the face, particularly with regard to forehead- and facelift techniques. He has been doing pioneering work in the field of aesthetic surgery for years: he was the first specialist in Switzerland to practise aesthetic surgery mainly on an outpatient basis or with a minimal stay in a clinic and to perform facial surgery exclusively under local anaesthesia and sedation. In 1990 he established his own clinic, the Burki Clinic for Aesthetic Surgery, which was one of the first in Europe to specialize primarily in aesthetic facial surgery. Urs Victor Burki has also broken new ground in terms of patient information. For more than ten years he has been providing his patients with detailed information, not only by richly illustrated brochures describing the main points of the surgical aspects, preoperative considerations and postoperative care, but also by using video films showing operating techniques and patient interviews.

Ever since he embarked on his professional career, one of Urs Victor Burki's main concerns has been to raise constantly the quality of aesthetic surgery through ongoing specific training and in-service training. That is why he founded the Swiss Society for Aesthetic Surgery (SSAS) in 1994, of which I am a founding member.

I can recommend not only the public at large but also all physicians to read this extensive and very artistically designed book.

Leo Clodius

Former professor of the Plastic, Reconstructive and Aesthetic Surgery Department at the University Hospital of Zurich. Former president of the Swiss Society for Plastic, Reconstructive and Aesthetic Surgery. Lecturer at the University of Zurich. Certified by the American Board of Plastic Surgery

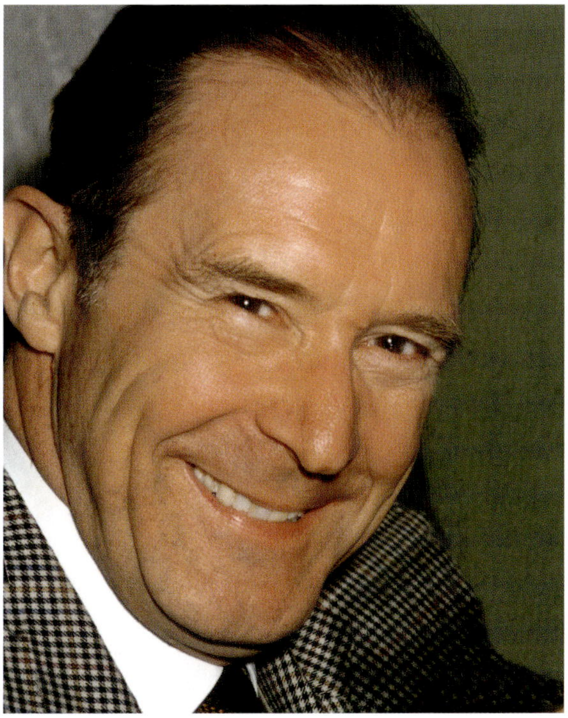

Prof. Leo Clodius, M.D.

"Quod est maius mirabile (...)? Diversitas et excellentia facierum: inter tot enim homines, qui fuerunt ab initio mundi et usque in finem futuri sunt, duo reperiri non possent, quorum facies per omnia similes sint vel possent."

"Which is the greatest marvel (...)? the diversity and excellence of the faces of men: for among all so many men as have been sith the beginning of the world unto the end, two men might not be found of whom their faces were like and semblable in all things."

Jacobus de Voragine (1230–1298)

From:
The Golden Legend or Lives of the Saints
Compiled by Jacobus de Voragine, archbishop of Genoa, 1275, first edition 1470
English version by William Caxton,
first edition 1483
From the Temple Classics, volume two, The Life of St. Andrew, edited by F. S. Ellis, 1900, page 42

Introduction

Occasionally dazzling under the media spotlights, but imperfectly revealed, aesthetic surgery fascinates. Every new technique - the latest way of improving a person's looks and warding off the ravages of age - captures our attention. But what is the real value of aesthetic surgery? What should we expect of it? A new technique is not validated just because it has been featured on television or a magazine has praised its merits. Nothing actually confirms that it has been tested by responsible aesthetic surgeons.

In recent years amazing progress has been made in aesthetic surgery of the face. Modern, less invasive operating techniques allow for better and longer-lasting results and make it possible to reduce considerably the post-operative recovery period. These operating procedures include primarily forehead and eyebrow lifts carried out with endoscopic technology. The preferred method of anaesthesia in facial aesthetic surgery today is no longer general, but local anaesthesia in combination with more or less deep sedation. Most experienced specialists currently employ this milder anaesthetic technique for all facial aesthetic operations, to the great satisfaction of their patients.

This book provides answers to questions that may be raised by a specific aesthetic procedure on the face; it describes the various surgical techniques as well as the pre- and postoperative considerations. It offers not only a panorama of aesthetic surgery's achievements, but also aids comprehension of the limitations of this surgical speciality. Clearly, such a book cannot substitute for the dialogue established between an experienced aesthetic surgeon and his or her patient. On the contrary, the pages in this book about the different aesthetic procedures on the face will facilitate that dialogue and will allow the interested reader to gain a clearer understanding of the options afforded by proven techniques.

Many years' practice in aesthetic surgery has confirmed my belief that proper patient information is essential. When patients consult a surgeon, they do not confine their questions to operating techniques; they seek a much more global enquiry, their concerns are much more general. Aesthetic choices as well as the status and social legitimacy of a particular notion of beauty are questions which must be addressed before an operation is considered.

Aesthetic surgery blends art with science. For this reason I am presenting aesthetic surgery of the face not only as a purely medical, but also as an artistic science, ultimately guided by the quest for harmony. In the course of many years of research on the natural laws that underly beauty and harmony of forms, I have studied the theories of proportion elaborated by Albrecht Dürer and Leonardo da Vinci. They inspired me to conduct in-depth studies of the facial proportions. In this book I describe in detail the insights I have gained.

Moreover, since my personal interests have led me to broaden my field of investigation in the quest of beauty through art and philosophy, I feel that a book such as this can also stimulate the reflection of all who are involved with the question of aesthetics. As I will demonstrate, beauty is not an unequivocal, established standard, but a phenomenon that encompasses an individual's sense of harmony and well-being.

Why focus exclusively on the face? There are two reasons. First, we are witnessing currently a process of specialization within the discipline itself. Since this book is confined to facial aesthetic surgery, it offers a review of the principal procedures in that area. Secondly, the face is proverbially a "mirror of the soul" and in that sense it requires the greatest care and attention.

Leonardo da Vinci – a Rich Source of Inspiration

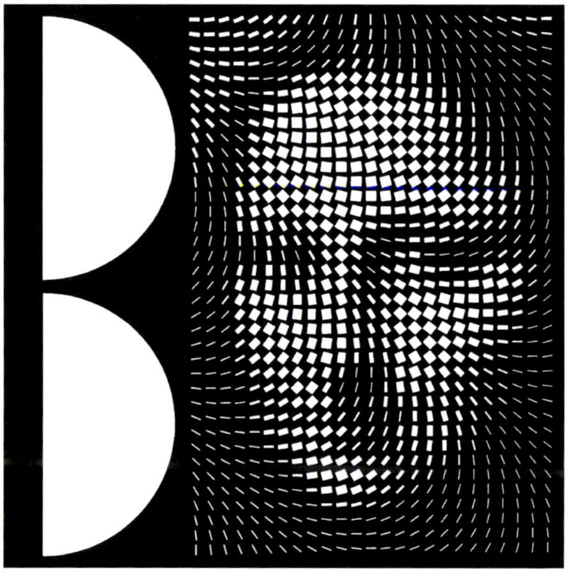

1

The universal genius, Leonardo da Vinci (1452-1519), bequeathed to humanity more than five thousand pages of manuscripts. Ever since I began my university studies I have concerned myself time and again with these documents.

The body of thought of the genius scientist and artist has influenced my work as an aesthetic surgeon in diverse ways.

Leonardo da Vinci's life work gives us an insight into a scientific way of looking at the human being, an approach that is based on a great knowledge of natural laws. In addition to his tireless research in the various fields of the natural sciences and technology, he was one of the first artists to study the proportions of the human body in all its detail. His most important contribution to the field of anatomy was the systematic and precise description of the human body. His tireless creative mind was driven by a desire to probe the "causal aspect" concealed behind natural phenomena.

This holistic approach is also reflected in his painting. According to the French lyric poet Paul Valéry (1871–1945), who was fascinated by the work of this great master, Leonardo regarded painting as a philosophy and used it as an instrument in his efforts to probe the mysteries of the universe. Johann Wolfgang von Goethe

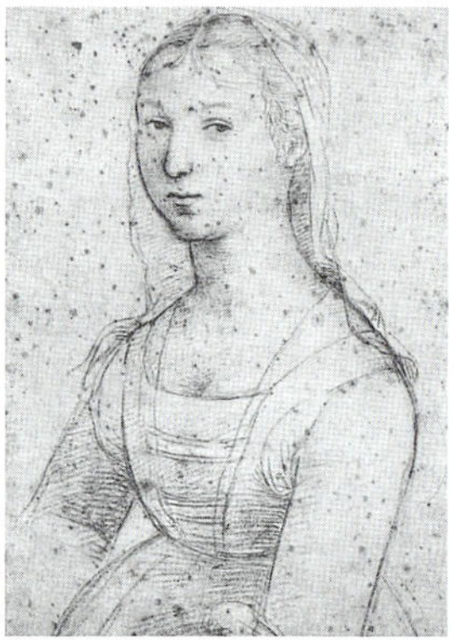

2

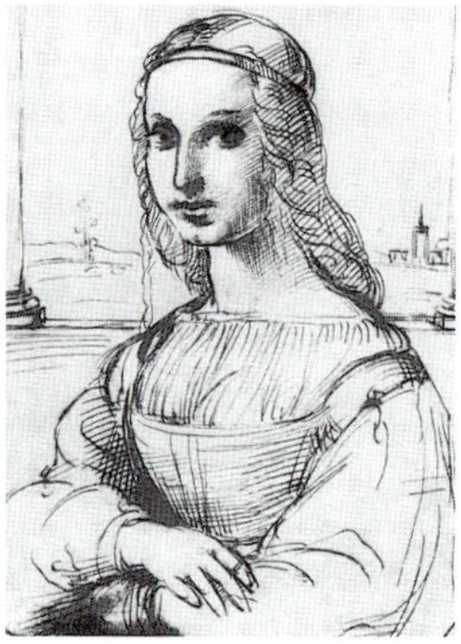

3

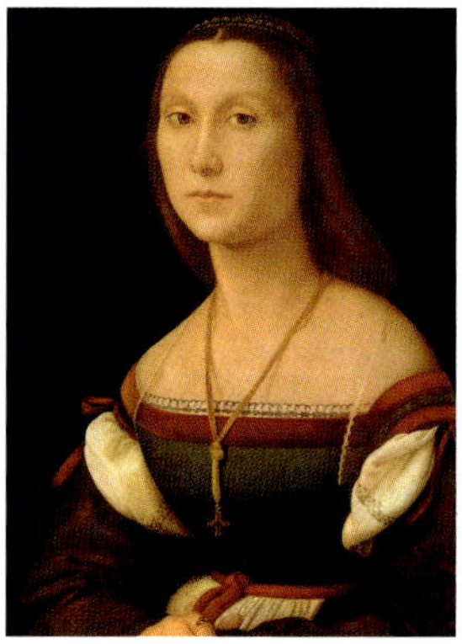

4

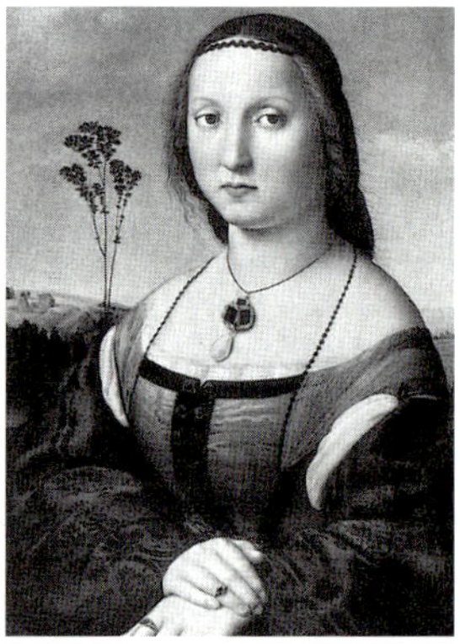

5

1 Logo of the Burki Clinic for Aesthetic Surgery created by Yvaral, son of Victor Vasarely, from the painting Mona Lisa synthétisée ML 266, 259x175cm, 1985, Yvaral. Collection Burki Clinic for Aesthetic Surgery, Geneva

2 Raphael, Woman's portrait, British Museum, London

3 Raphael, Woman's portrait, The Louvre, Paris

4 Raphael, Woman's portrait, called The Dumb Woman, Galleria Nazionale delle Marche, Urbino

5 Raphael, Portrait of Maddalena Doni, Palatina Gallery, Florence

6 Leonardo da Vinci, the Mona Lisa, The Louvre, Paris

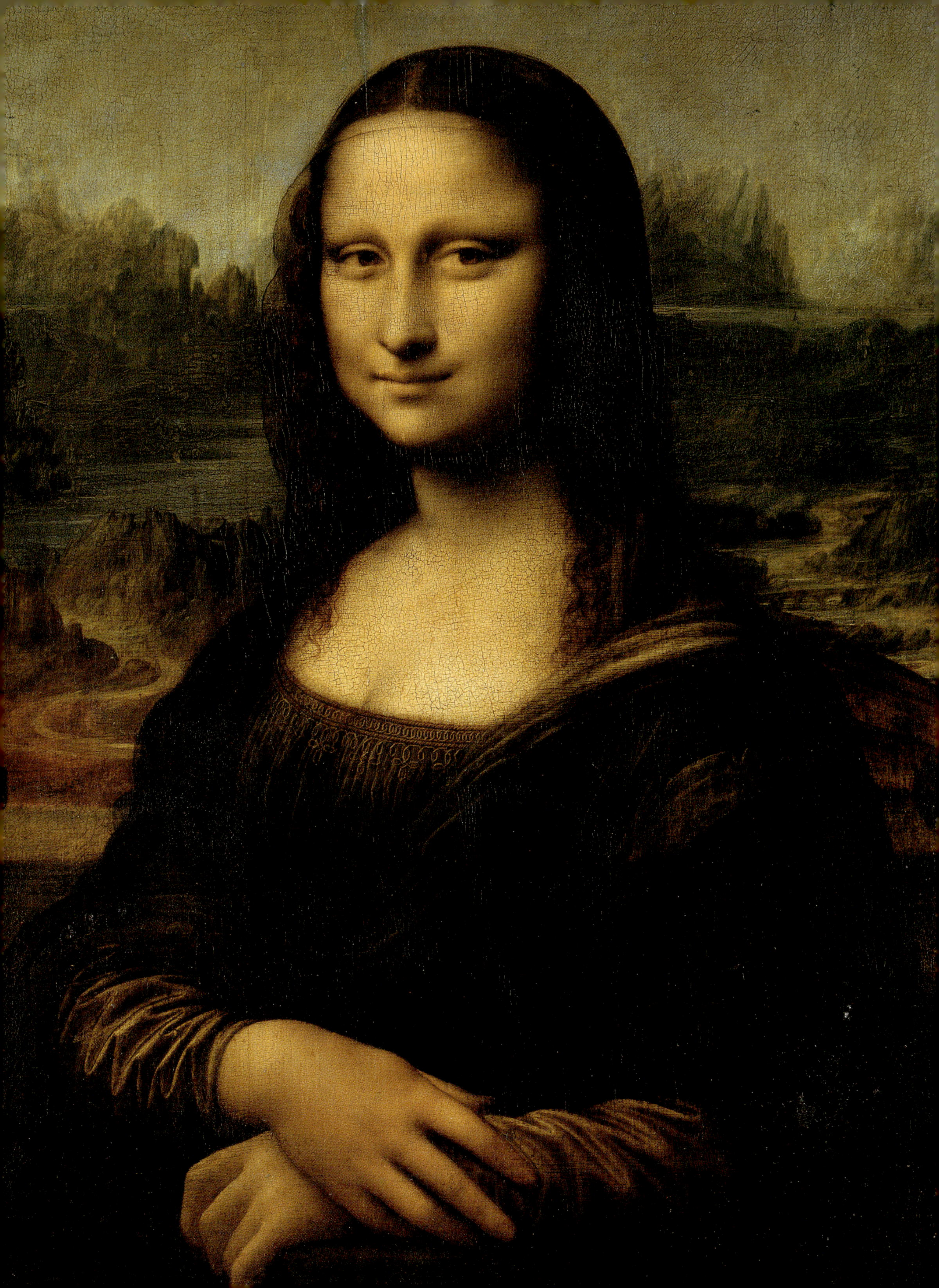

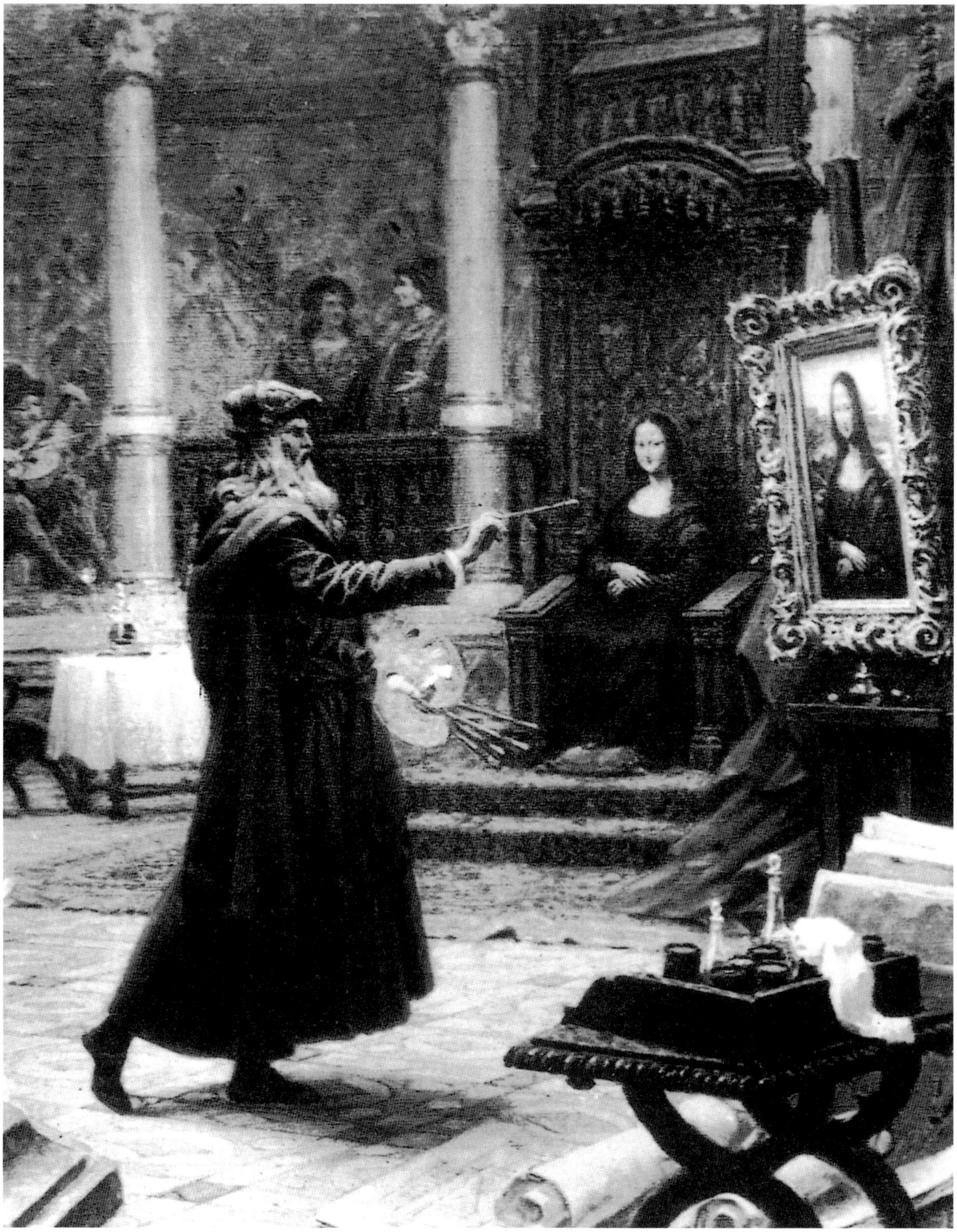

7

7 L. Béroud, Leonardo da Vinci and the Mona Lisa (Salon, 1920). Collection Roger-Viollet, Paris

(1741–1832) commented on Leonardo da Vinci during one of his journeys to Italy as follows, "... he did not rely on the inner drive of his innate, inestimable talent, no arbitrary, chance flash of inspiration was to prevail, everything had to be carefully considered and reflected on."[1]

In his Treatise on Painting *(Trattato Della Pittura)* Leonardo da Vinci recorded for the artists of his time many precepts, which he also followed in his own creative work. In Leonardo's view, the supreme art of painting was not merely to portray the appearance but also the emotions of the model. "Essentially, a good painter should reveal two things: the image of man and the essence of his mind. The first is easy, the second difficult..."[2] For Leonardo, investigating the visible world was a way of capturing supernatural reality that was imbued with the soul. "If you think his physical constitution is a marvel of skill, it is nothing in comparison with the spirit that resides in such a structure."[3] The ideas that he records in his treatise on painting about his artistic ideals were my gateway to his intellectual world, which is uniquely expressed in his works of art.

Leonardo's ideal of beauty is expressed in many of his paintings. For example, in the portrait *the Musician, the Lady with an Ermine* and *the Belle Ferronière* (see chapter on *Ideals of Beauty and Facial Proportions*, figs. 19, 21, 22). We find the ideal of the radiant portrait, in which outer and inner beauty combine, in the mysterious countenance of the Mona Lisa (fig. 6). If one contemplates this world-famous painting intensively, one is transported almost magically into a world linked to the most profound part of our being. It is this inspired aura that is expressed in the mysterious smile of the Gioconda (Mona Lisa) that fascinates people of all cultures time and again. The Mona Lisa, more than any other portrait, has inspired many important artists to do their own interpretations, from Raphael to Yvaral (figs. 1–5). Leonardo da Vinci is thought to have begun this masterpiece in Florence at the age of 47 and to have completed it three years later in 1506. This painting, which was never handed over to the person who commissioned it, remained in Leonardo's possession for the rest of his life. In 1515 he took it with him to the estate of King Francis the First's castle at Amboise-on-the-Loire, the master's last residence. According to the historian, painter and architect Giorgio Vasari (1511–1574), Mona Lisa - which is an abbreviation of Madonna Lisa - was the third wife of a Florentine merchant by the name of Francesco Bartolomeo del Giocondo; hence the name La Gioconda. She is said to have been about twenty-four years old when Leonardo painted her portrait for the first time.

In his famous biographies of artists' lives, Vasari described how the portrait of the Mona Lisa originated. Leonardo da Vinci went so far in his quest for perfection that he had singers and musicians come and entertain his model by playing the lute, singing songs and telling amusing stories (fig. 7). Vasari wrote: "...the smile on this face is so lovely that it is heavenly rather than earthly."[4]

Perhaps if Leonardo da Vinci were living today he would be among the most gifted of aesthetic surgeons. With his medical background, aesthetic temperament and eye for beauty he possessed the virtues which have inspired me in my practice and endeavour to create artful results on the canvas of the human face.

[1] *Mario Pomillo, Leonardo da Vinci, die Klassiker der Kunst, Editions Rizzoli, Milan, 1967, p. 10*

[2] *Heinrich Ludwig, Leonardo da Vinci, das Buch von der Malerei, Wilhelm Braumüller, Vienna, 1882, p. 128,*

[3] *Woldemar von Seidlitz, Leonardo da Vinci, der Wendepunkt der Renaissance, Editions Phaidon, Vienna, 1935, p. 409 (l. 1140)*

[4] *Giorgio Vasari, Lebensläufe, Leonardo da Vinci, Editions Manesse, Zurich, 1974, p. 33*

Mona Lisa –
her Aesthetic Operation

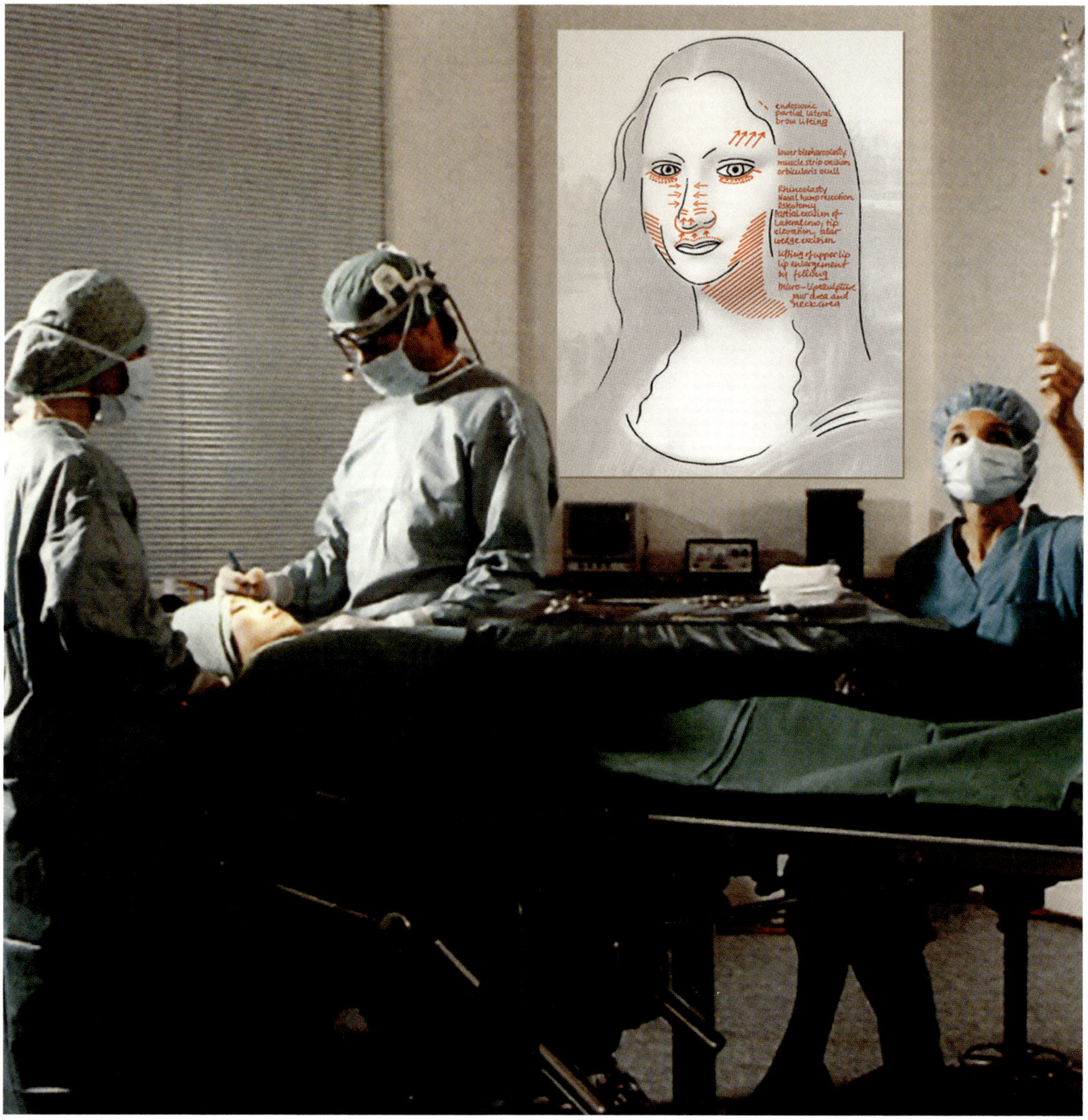

1

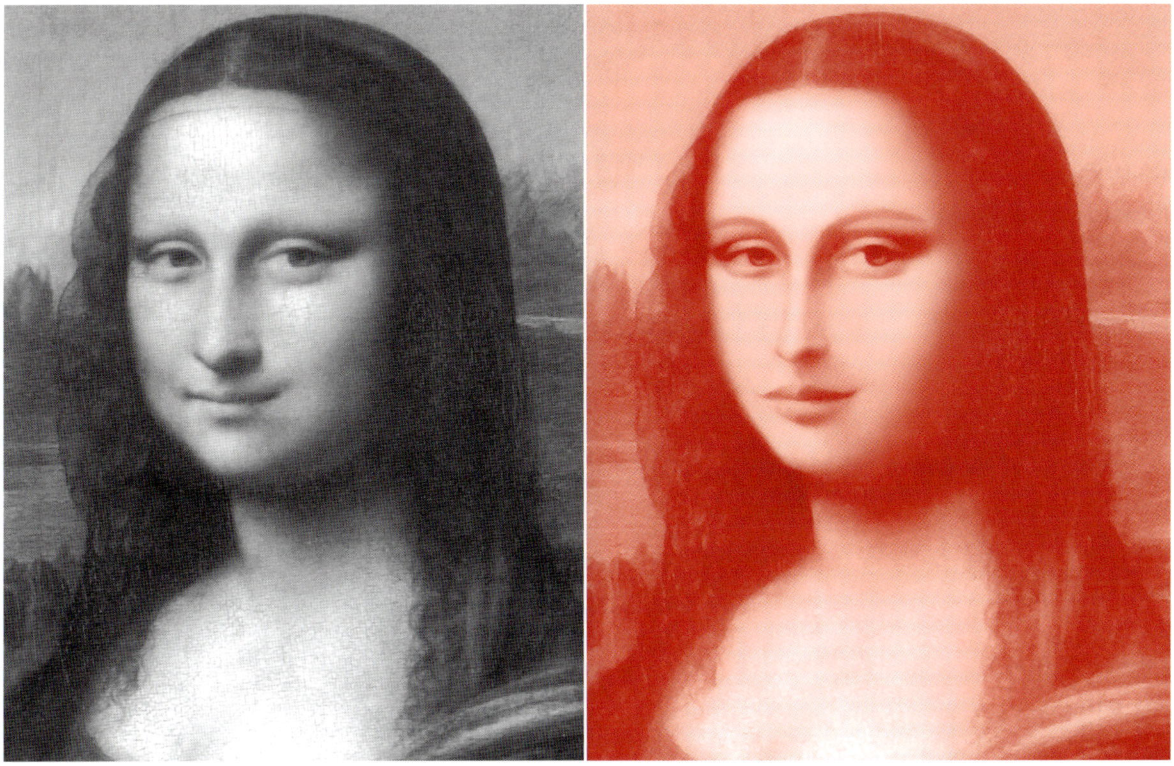

2

The Mona Lisa by Leonardo da Vinci has been described countless times as the mirror image of the master's soul. The portrait has fascinated me since my early youth and it is constantly on my mind. I too have been captivated by her aura and she has never released me. Mona Lisa's enigmatic smile and her captivating gaze attract hundreds of thousands of visitors from all over the world to The Louvre every year. The Mona Lisa is thus today the emblem of my clinic.

This world-famous painting has inspired many important artists to create their own interpretations. Recently, when studying intensively the proportions of the human face as drawn by Leonardo da Vinci and comparing carefully the proportions of Mona Lisa's face, the mysterious woman – now more than five hundred years old – revealed herself as in a dream: I was performing an aesthetic operation on Mona Lisa's face in a baroque period concert hall, to the accompaniment of organ music. The images of this dream haunted me obsessively, and I pondered how to alter her face to bring her closer to today's ideal of beauty. I decided to turn the dream into reality and to proceed with an actual aesthetic operation on Mona Lisa in my Clinic. The result of this train of reflections is expressed in figures 2–4, which show the specific operating techniques used. The alterations made correspond to the criteria of beauty valid today. By way of clarification: the result was by no means obtained by using a computer, nor was it done at my own discretion or merely as I thought. Rather I proceeded as if Mona Lisa were my patient. In order to achieve the result shown, I decided in favour of operating techniques that are technically feasible and that make sense in the light of current scientific knowledge. (figs. 3a–d)

1 Imaginary aesthetic operation of Mona Lisa

2 Mona Lisa before/after the aesthetic operation. Conception: Urs Victor Burki.

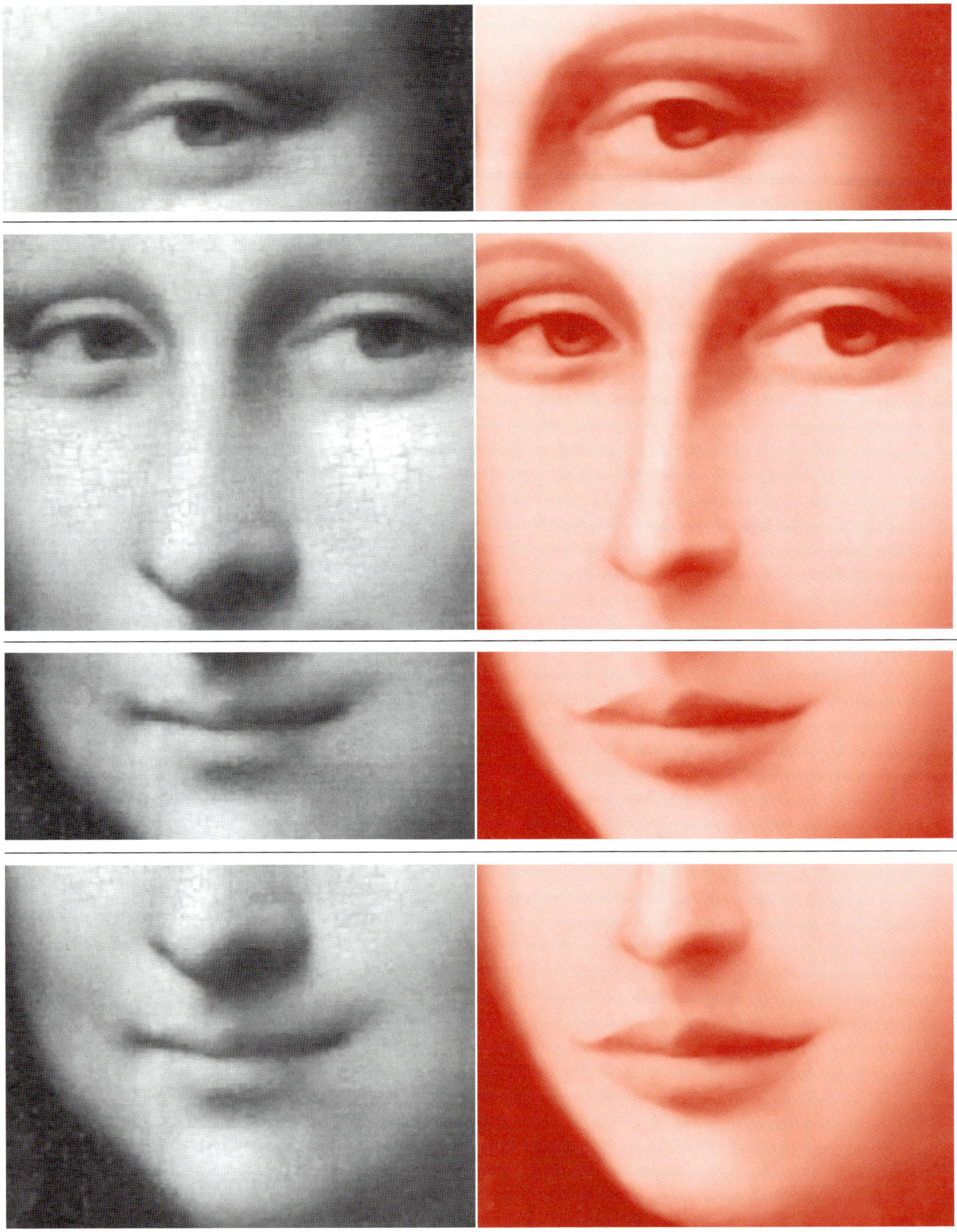

3a,b,c,d

Forehead/Eyes: Lifting of the temporal region with a slight raising of the outer part of the eyebrows. Lower eyelid plasty with a slight excision of the orbicularis muscle (fig. 3a).

Nose: Aesthetic rinoplasty. Removal of the bony and cartilaginous hump, osteotomy to narrow the nose, excision of the cephalic part of the alar cartilage to reduce the size of the nasal tip and to create a more harmonious tip-contour. To achieve a narrower tip, the alar cartilage on the dome is weakened by micro-incisions. A small amount of cartilage of the lower part of the septum is removed to improve the angle between upper lip and base of the nose (fig. 3b).

Lips: Lifting of the upper lip by skin excision on the base of the nose and the nostrils to enlarge the vermilion of the upper lip in proportion to the lower lip, enlargement of the upper and lower lip by filling (fig. 3c).

Face/Neck: Micro-liposculpture in the lower cheek, lower jaw and neck region to improve the contour of the lower face and neck (fig. 3d).

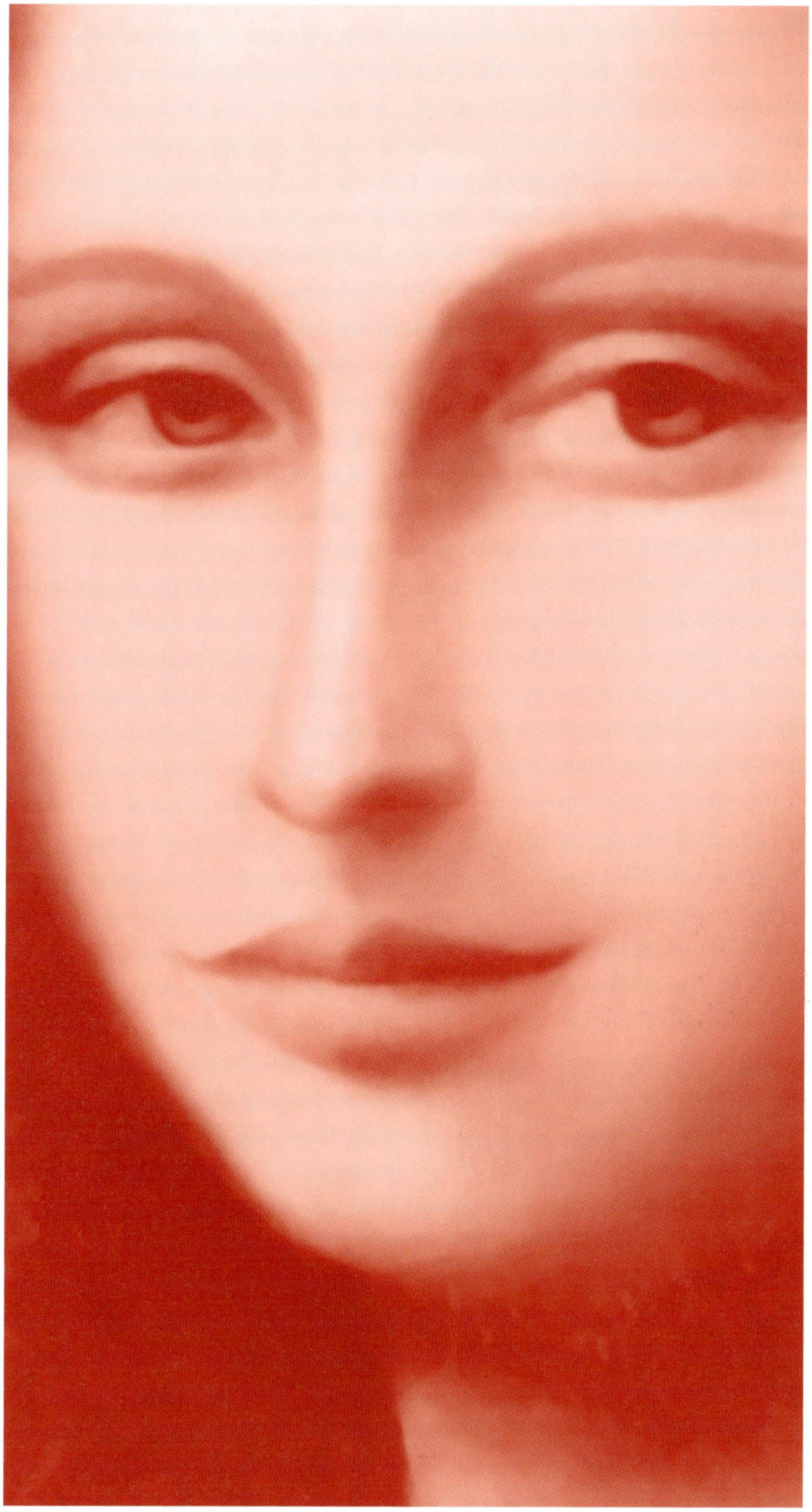

4

3 Surgical procedures and results in the different regions of the face: a) forehead/eyes, b) nose, c) lips, d) face/neck
4 Mona Lisa after the aesthetic operation. Conception: Urs Victor Burki.

The Quest for Beauty

Man's quest for beauty probably first took on meaning when he observed his image on the surface of water – his first mirror. When Narcissus discovered himself – as a moving reflection on a blue surface, it was not so much what we now incorrectly call narcissism that caused him to marvel, but much more the revelation of his own deep-seated identity sculpted in his features. Imagine walking along the edge of an expanse of water and, attracted by its unfathomable and mysterious depths, you lower your face to within a few inches of the surface. The mystery of your face is suddenly revealed to you; for the first time you see what others see. And moreover: you observe how your features reveal the joy and sadness you feel, register surprise at what you see and translate what you hear.

Ever since the most ancient civilizations human beings have used all the means at their disposal to adapt their appearance to the current criteria of beauty. Such ideals not only differed from one culture to another, they also remained subject to change over time within a particular culture. Despite the existence of fundamental universal criteria beauty isn't a quality in things themselves, it exists merely in the mind which contemplates them and each mind perceives a different beauty. However, our perception of beauty is largely determined by aesthetic and social trends.

In the many ages of civilization great artists have expressed the ideals of beauty (figs. 1–8). The world-famous bust of the Egyptian queen and wife of Amenophis IV, Nofretete, created by Thutmosis of Achet-Aton, embodies an ideal of beauty passed on to the subsequent generations (fig. 1). Nofretete (in ancient Egyptian "Ne-fer-tari", meaning "beauty has come") is still regarded as an ideal of beauty today, 3300 years after her death.

In ancient Egypt men and women used to attach great importance to their appearance. They used to lighten their facial skin with yellow and white pigments and in order to give their cheeks and lips a "healthy" colour, they painted them with ochre-coloured pigments. They underlined the contours of their eyes with a thin pencil using plenty of charcoal. Charcoal was also applied to shadow the eyelids. This characteristic make-up is expressed in many Egyptian sculptures (figs. 1–3). Then as today, make-up styles were dictated by fashion. When Cleopatra (69–30 BC), Queen of Egypt, decided to shade her upper eyelids dark blue and her lower eyelids light green and to apply green copper pigment to her lips, the ladies of the court followed her example.

The frequent depictions of valuable cosmetic utensils, mirrors, combs and cosmetic caskets in tomb paintings indicate the great value that was attached to cosmetics in ancient Egypt. Apart from decorative cosmetics, other methods and artifices were also used to embellish one's appearance or to conceal any blemishes. For example, Egyptian men used to make their skin tighter with astringent fluids. To eliminate wrinkles, they used to wear face masks of mixtures of alabaster, salt and honey. In addition, they used special fluids to remove pimples and warts.

Then as today, celebrations were a good opportunity to show oneself at one's best. On festive occasions Egyptian men and women used to cover up their everyday hairstyle with a wig. Portrayals of garments and archaeological discoveries of highly symbolic jewellery bear witness to the aristocratic elegance that prevailed in the kingdom of Pharaohs.

Beauty was also held in high esteem in ancient Greece. For the Greeks, it was a trait of one's personality, which earned respect and praise. Their

1 Nofretete, Egyptian Museum, State Museums, Berlin

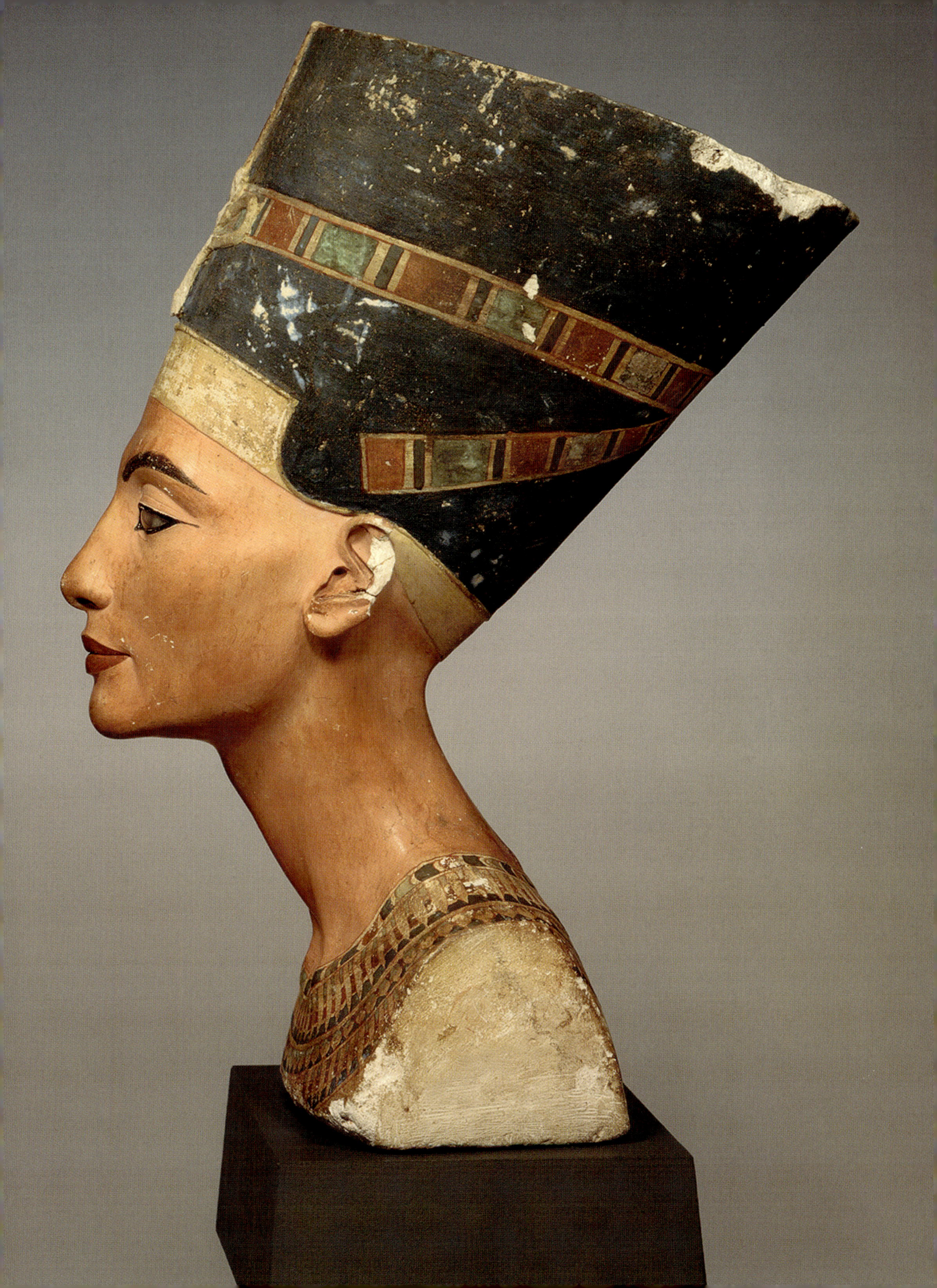

gods embodied ideal human figures. Among the Greeks, a perfectly formed body which captured people's attention with its absolutely harmonious proportions prompted a strong desire to strive to imitate the gods on Mount Olympus – at least in appearance. The gods were people's ideal of beauty. On their family altars stood statuettes of Aphrodite, the goddess of love and beauty, and of Apollo, the god of light and poetry. The purpose of these revered objects was to fuel the striving for perfection and to train the eye to recognize perfection. Inner and outer beauty were one in the minds of the Greeks and were expressed equally in painting and sculpture. Classical Antiquity's ideal of beauty is the expression of a philosophy of life characterized by the striving for order and harmony.

Cosmetic techniques in ancient Greece were not the preserve of the rich and powerful. The hetaerans – the ancient Greeks' courtesans – were extremely skilful at using cosmetics, unlike respectable Greek women. They covered their folds with a lead-containing paste, dyed their grey hairs or bleached them to obtain a blond tone. Hair was usually woven into neat plaits (fig. 5).

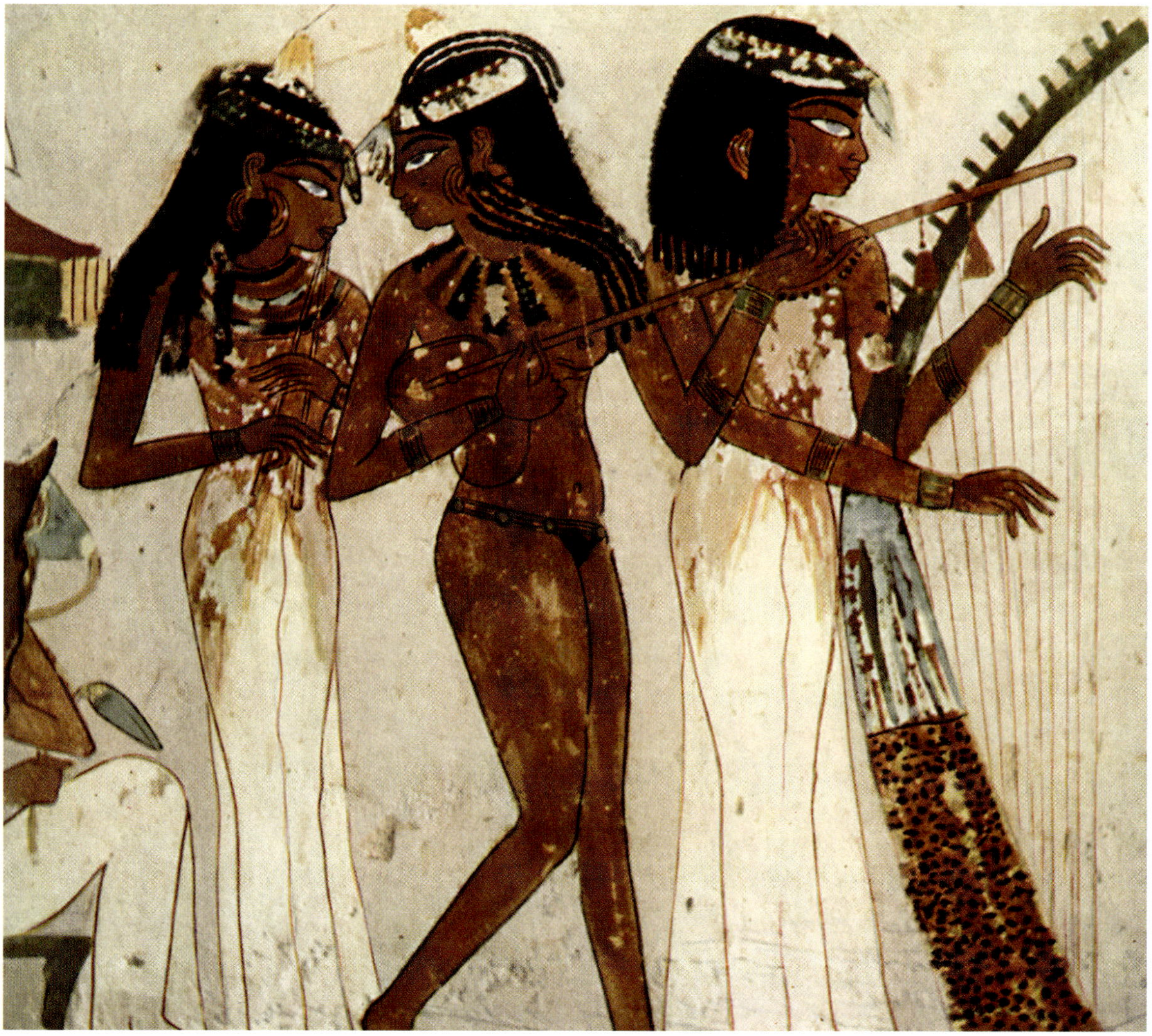

2

2 Fresco in the tomb of a priest of Amon in the reign of Amenophis II, Thebes

3 Queen Merit-Amon, Egyptian Museum, Cairo

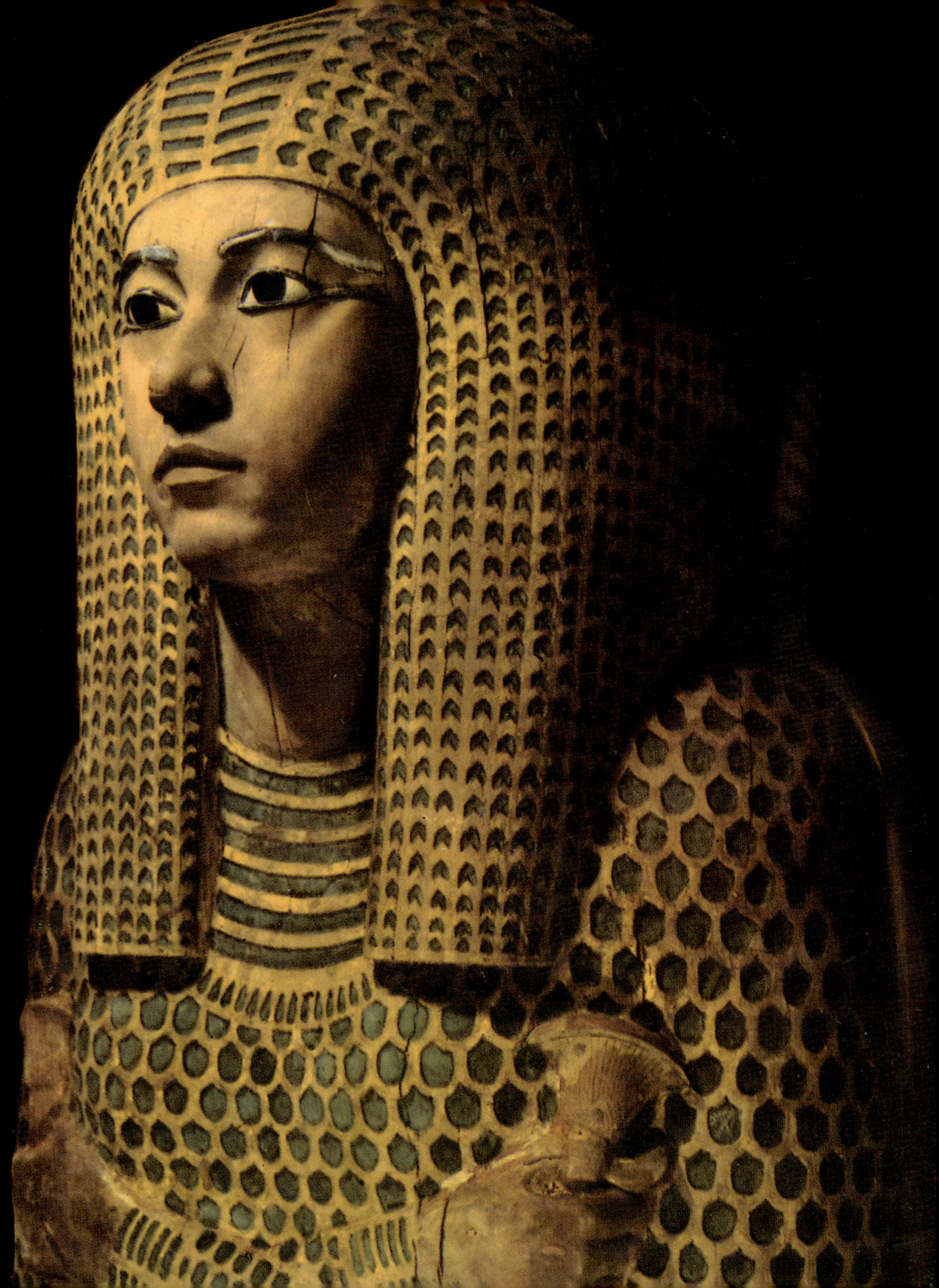

Black-contoured eyelids and black-dyed eyebrows were also in fashion.

Roman men also employed aids to beauty. Emperor Nero (37–68 AD), for example, used to bleach his face and body. Special attention was likewise paid to a beautiful hairstyle in Roman culture (figs. 6, 7). The visit to the hairdresser was a ritual. It was also very popular among Roman women to wear wigs. They spent much time attending to their hairstyle, making up their face, shading their eyebrows, eyelashes and lips, and used to purchase expensive gold, perfume and jewellery from distant lands (fig. 4). Men cared for their bodies by perspiring in public steam baths and having themselves massaged with precious oils.

In his treatise *Ars amatoria* (The Art of Love)[1], the Roman poet Publius Ovidius Naso, who is known as Ovid (43 BC-17/18 AD) gives women advice on the art of making themselves look their best. "Neatness is what we (men) like. Let your hair be nicely done."[2] One should choose a hairstyle that best suits the shape of one's face and suppresses the grey streaks that detract from general harmony: "A woman will dye her grey hair with the juice of some German herb; and the artificial colour becomes her better than the natural one."[3] Does she think her eyebrows are a little thin? All she need do is thicken them with a black powder or candle snuff. She should choose her clothes with care, because not all colours suit all people, and it is not advisable to wear "garments heavily inwrought with gold. "... the wealth by which you would fain attract us, very often just repels us".[4] Ovid considers that beauty care is very important for women. "Rare, however, is the face without a fault. Hide these blemishes with care, and so far as may be, conceal the defects of your figure."[5] Any woman can enhance her charms by bringing out the radiance of her complexion with powder, by masking the paleness of her face with purple vermilion and by underlining her eyes with finely powdered ash or a touch of Sicilian saffron. Nevertheless Ovid warns his lady readers: "But on no account let your lover find you with a

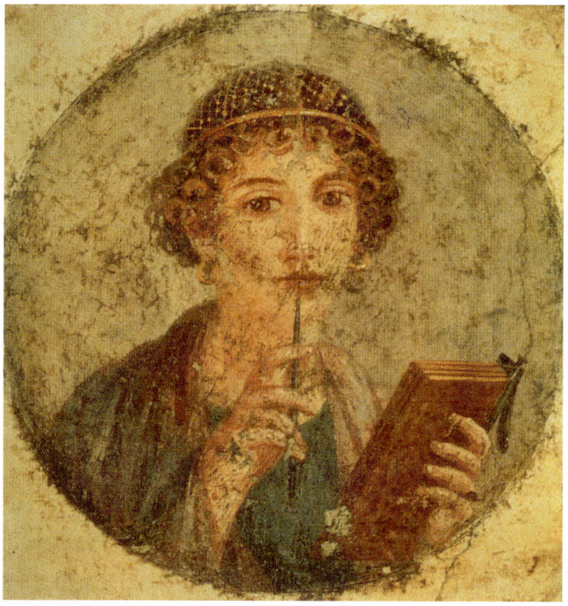

4

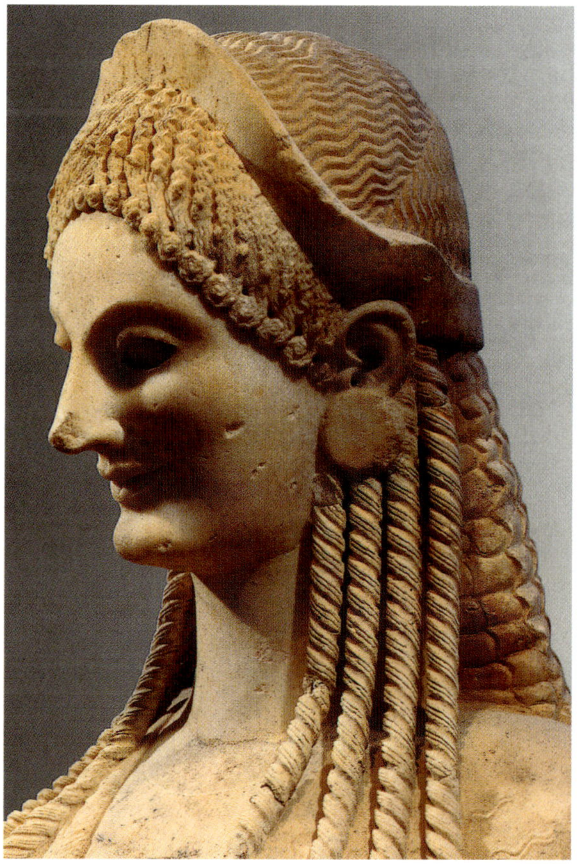

5

4 Woman's portrait, painted medallion, National Archaeological Museum, Naples
5 Kore, Acropolis of Athens

lot of 'aids to beauty' boxes about you. The art that adorns you should be unsuspected."[6] However, for the poet, all these artifices are merely the counterpart of a decent attitude and a pleasant personality. To keep one's good looks, one must learn to restrain one's temper: "Peace, gentle peace, is the attribute of man, as rage and fury are the characteristics of wild beasts."[7]. "You must have a soft, appealing expression, if you want to attract a lover."[8]

History is strewn with examples that testify to people's unceasing desire to alter their appearance. From the most ancient civilizations until modern times, humans have resorted to all kinds of methods to modify their features, thereby obeying the criteria of beauty set by society. Also aesthetic surgery of the face springs from man's need to express himself through his appearance. The quest for aesthetics and beauty is more than mere vanity: it is a primal human need, a perfectly legitimate desire for personal well-being. In 1930 Sigmund Freud stated: "Aesthetic pleasure, as a slightly inebriating emotion, has a special character. The utilitarian aspect of beauty does not appear clearly; one cannot discern that it is necessary to civilization, yet the latter would not be able to do without it."[9]

[1] *Ovid, Ars amatoria (The Art of Love), translated from the Latin by J. Lewis May, Rarity Press, New York, 1930*

[2-8] *Ovid, Ars 3, verses 133, 163-164, 132-133, 261-262, 208-209, 509, 510 in: op. cit.*

[9] *Sigmund Freud, Das Unbehagen in der Kultur (Civilization and its Discontents), 1930, in: Fragen der Gesellschaft, Ursprünge der Religion, Studienausgabe vol. IX, Suhrkamp, Frankfurt am Main, 1974, p. 214*

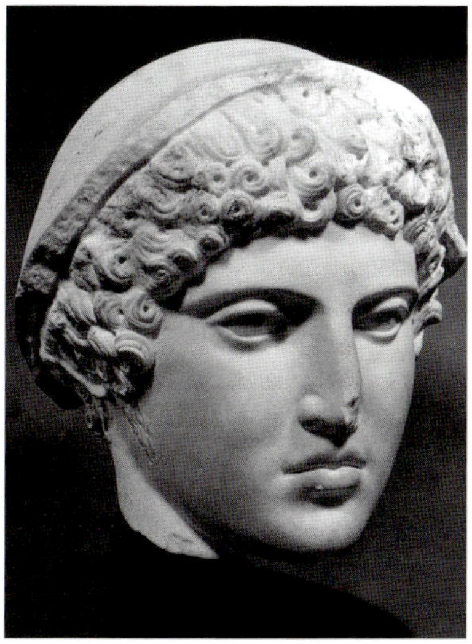

6

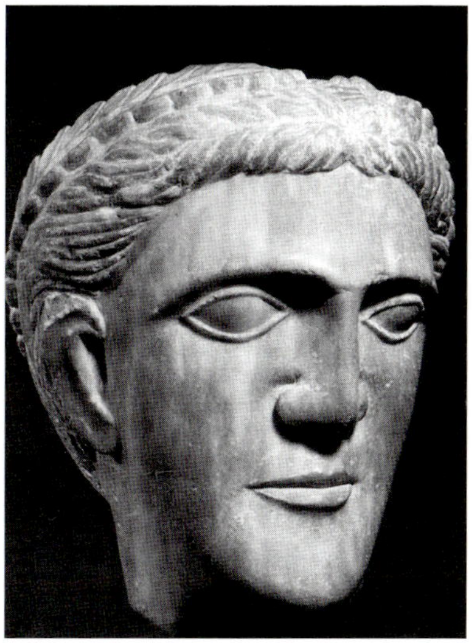

7

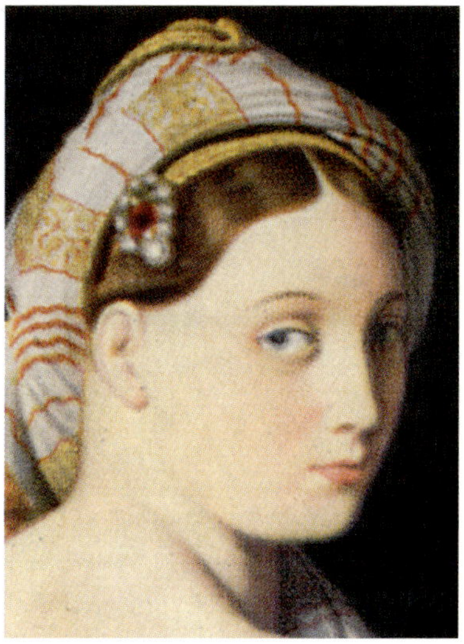

8

6 Hermes, 1st century, Private collection, in: Antikes Erbe, Orell Füssli, Zurich, 1965

7 Head, late Roman period, R. Schmidt collection, Solothurn, in: Antikes Erbe, Orell Füssli, Zurich, 1965

8 Jean-Auguste-Dominique Ingres, reclining odalisque known as "Grand Odalisque", The Louvre, Paris

Beauty – in the Eyes of the Philosophers

In western culture the concept of beauty finds its true origins in the fifth and sixth centuries BC, in the age of classical Greece and the hegemony of Athens. After conquering the great Persian Empire, Athens became a flourishing intellectual and cultural centre. From Pericles to the conquests of Alexander the Great, the theory of the beautiful and the aesthetic reached its apogee there, and it was to be several centuries before any new ideas emerged.

From the Pythagoreans of the fifth century BC we inherited a definition of beauty which was widely embraced in the whole of Antiquity. For the followers of Pythagoras (580–497 BC; fig. 1), the state of being beautiful is defined by number and measurement. Beauty is the very essence of order; it reflects the objective quality of things, that is, *harmonia* (order and concordance of elements), and *symmetria* (correct proportions that conform to the measurement).

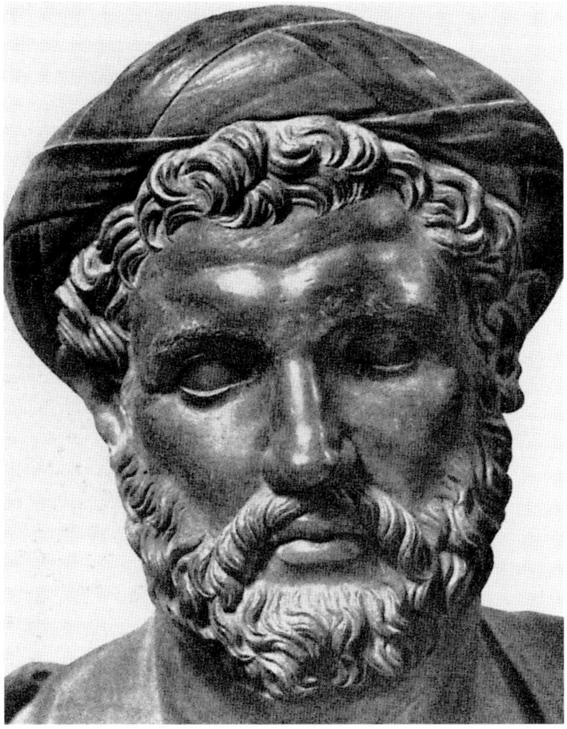

1

Conversely, the Sophists adopted a relativist view of beauty, relying on Protagoras's celebrated adage: "Man (that is, every being taken individually) is the measure of all things." According to this perspective, only subjective perception – each person's taste – is capable of defining what is beautiful. What pleases the eye or ear is beautiful. But such a denial of objectivity was not acceptable to everybody – indeed it was passionately opposed by Plato and Aristotle.

Plato (427–347 BC; fig. 3) ventured to give various definitions of the beautiful in his dialogues that took the form of aphorisms (cf. in *Phaidros* and *Symposion*, in connection with the notions of the divine, of good and wisdom): he espoused the dimension of the "sensually pleasing" introduced by the Sophists in their approach to the concept, as well as the presumed position of Socrates, who regarded the beautiful as a practical and useful element, as radiance and light, a generator of the good and of perfection. It is certainly in *Hippias major* that the difficulty of explaining the notion of beauty presents itself most vividly. Plato has Socrates ask the Sophist Hippias to define beauty. The latter evades the question; he lists a series of objects representing that quality: a beautiful girl, a beautiful horse, a beautiful lyre. Feeling vexed, Socrates (470–399 BC; fig. 2) retorts that he does not want to know what he,

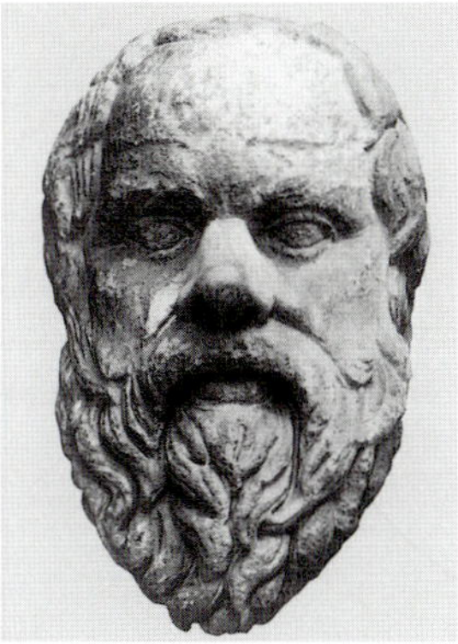

2

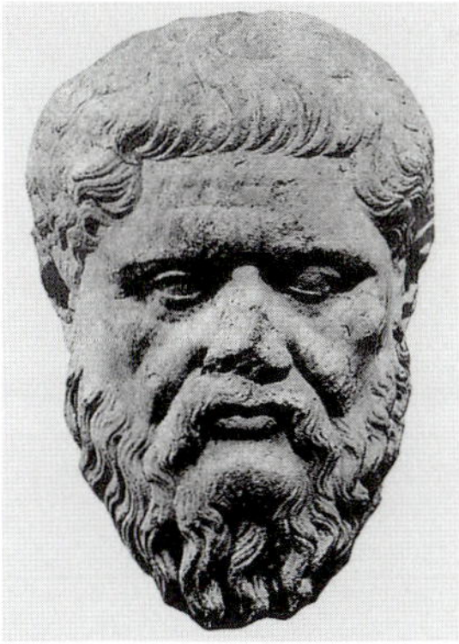

3

Hippias, considers or perceives to be beautiful, but "what beauty actually is". With Plato, the notion of beauty or the beautiful became a genuine philosophical problem. Far from being characteristic of objects in themselves, beauty should be sought in the quality that is the common denominator of beautiful objects. Socrates ends by admitting that it is impossible to answer this question. Moreover, how to identify this common denominator is still at the heart of the debate on beauty, even today.

With Aristotle (384–322 BC; fig. 4), beauty again became a quality distributed equally and objectively among works of art and natural objects. Their general forms are said to be order, harmony and precision (according to the Pythagorean tradition), as the mathematical sciences (metaphysics) demonstrate.

It was not until the neo-Platonism of the third century after Christ that the Platonic doctrine of beauty was revived, although it was modified in the light of Aristotelian ideas. This is borne out by Plotinus (203–269 AD; fig. 5), whose treatise "On Beauty" is his most famous work. Beauty is created with the generative power of the form emanating from the Gods. All things in the physical world are beautiful to the extent that they are imbued with this form. Moreover, the beautiful and the good are identical. The other type of beauty, which manifests itself in actions, originates from the creative soul. It is the soul that helps to make bodies beautiful because it is of divine essence and constitutes, as it were, a part of the beautiful.

Saint Augustine (354–430 AD; fig. 6) together with Plotinus agreed that the beautiful is identified by intelligence and not by the senses. The rational criteria that determine sensual beauty are equality and proportion, without which nothing truly beautiful can exist.

Saint Thomas Aquinas (1225–1274; fig. 7) re-established the importance of symmetry, order and proportion. According to him, beauty requires three elements: first of all, integrity or perfection *(integritas sive perfectio)*; then the right proportion or concordance *(debita proportio sive consonantia)* and finally clarity *(claritas)*. These definitions are the pillars on which the mediaeval doctrine of beauty rested: perfection, proportion and light, where the good and the

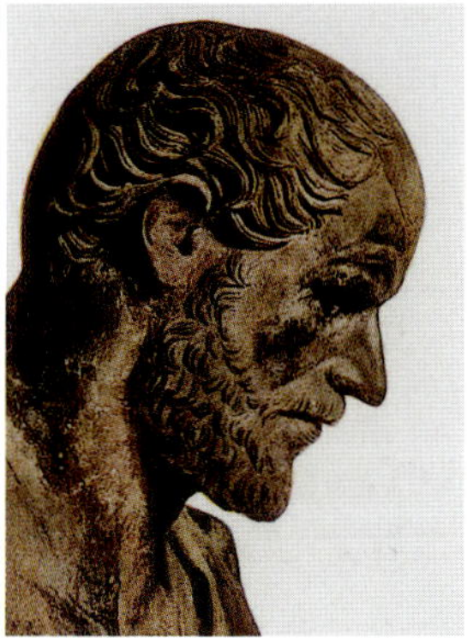

4

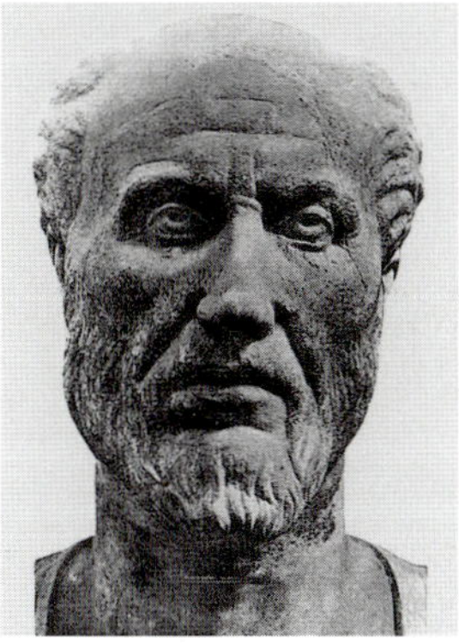

5

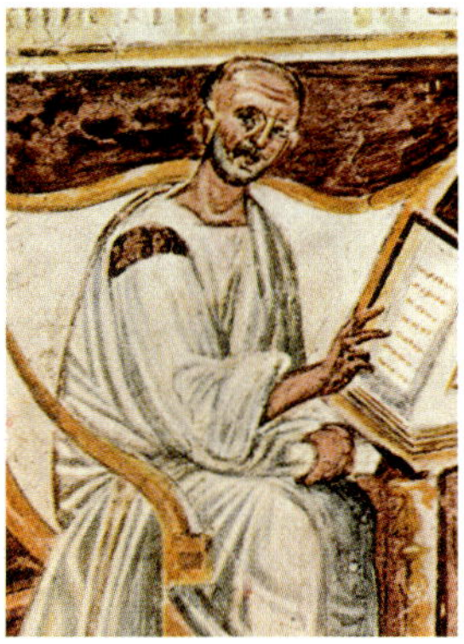

6

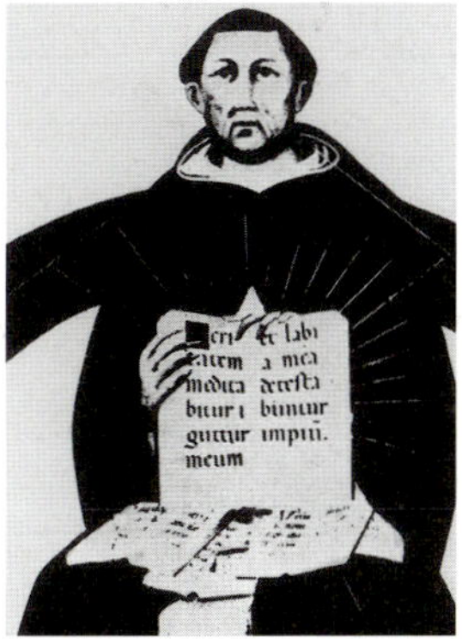

7

1 Pythagoras, bronze head, National Museum, Naples

2 Socrates, British Museum, London

3 Plato, National Museum, Athens

4 Aristotle, National Museum, Athens

5 Plotinus, Vatican Museums, Rome

6 Saint Augustine, mosaic, in: La saggezza dell'occidente, Longanesi, Milan, 1961

7 Saint Thomas Aquinas, The Vatican Library, Rome

beautiful are but one in material terms; at the conceptual level, however, they are different. One seeks to gain possession of the good, while one is content simply to look at the beautiful. *Pulchra enim dicantur quae visa placent*: the beautiful is described as what delights the eyes.

Brought up in the Platonic tradition, the philosopher Marsilio Ficino (1433–1499; fig. 8), a protégé of Prince Cosimo de Medicis, introduced a new element: beauty is the divine light that radiates from objects. In other words, the beauty of the world is founded on the way in which God seeks, through his love, to create a link between his creatures and himself, be they animate or not. By way of another original conclusion, Ficino suggests that the beauty of an object is gauged by the eye, not by the touch, and that consequently the object is brought to life not as such, but as an image. Thus it is not the object considered, but rather the image one has of it that is described as beautiful.

We owe two important treatises to the Scottish philosopher Francis Hutcheson (1694–1746; fig. 9) *An Inquiry into the Original of our Ideas of Beauty and Virtue*. For Hutcheson, the experience of beauty is a particular feeling of joy, which differs from other feelings in that it occurs directly, without the object being identified or without any reference to an expected utility or moral value. It is an almost instinctive and innate feeling. Since the phenomenon also applies to the external perceptive senses, the ability to experience beauty can be called a "sense". However, because this sense focuses not only on the object but well beyond - on the intelligible (for example, moral principles) - it is preferable to speak of it as an inner sense. The purpose of life is happiness, and for Hutcheson happiness resides in the experience of beauty. A beauty that is sensed, felt and conceptualized from experience, but that cannot be explained.

A few years later Bishop George Berkeley (1685–1753; fig. 10) declared that beauty, whether it be moral or sensorial in nature, can only be identified by reason; because the beauty of each object depends on the purpose assigned to it. The beautiful is always what is most suitable, be it in dress, architecture or any other expression.

Closer to our own times, in his book *A Philosophical Enquiry into the Origin of our Ideas of the Sublime and Beautiful*, the British writer Edmund Burke (1729–1797; fig. 11) refutes the idea that the beauty of an object lies entirely in its proportions. He observes that persons whose facial beauty is indisputable and acknowledged vary widely in their proportions. Conversely, perfect proportions are no guarantee of beauty, because the same proportions that determine the relationship between the facial features (nose, eyes, ears, etc.) and characterize a strikingly beautiful face do not always produce a beautiful person. The qualities truly capable of making an object appear to be beautiful are apprehended nei-

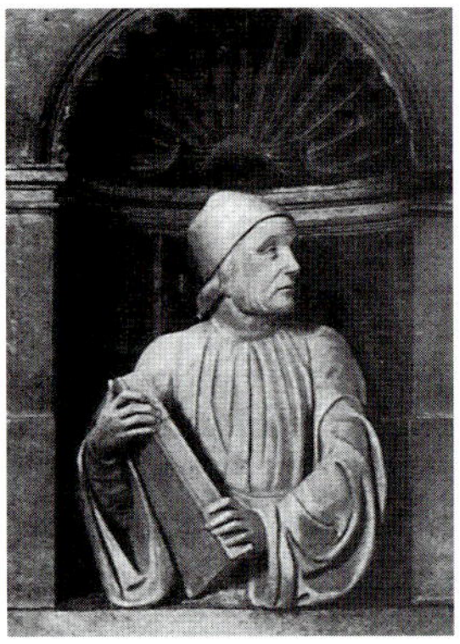

8

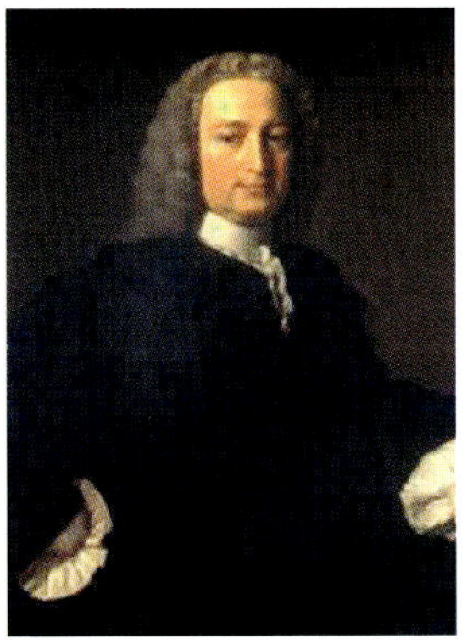

9

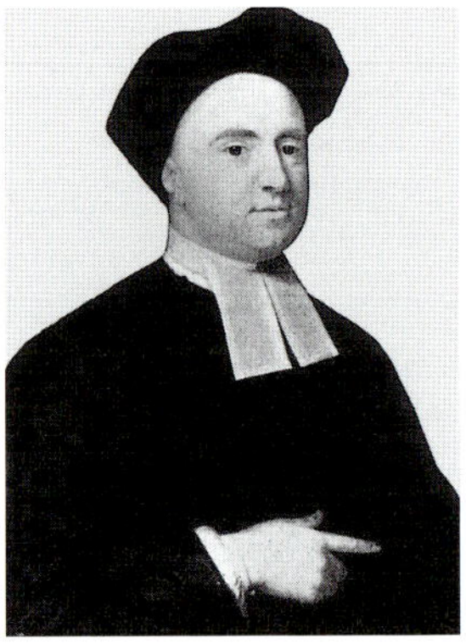

10

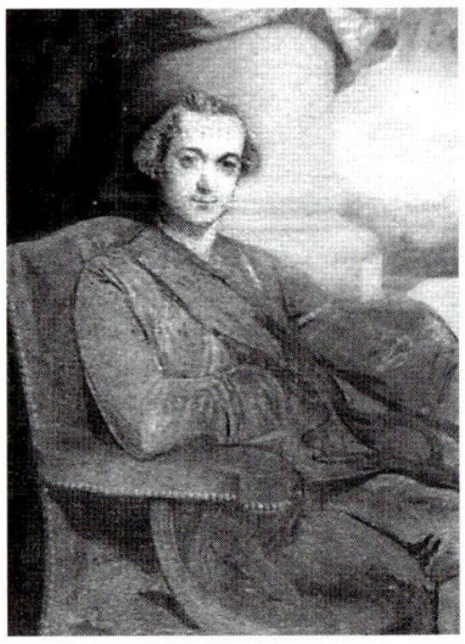

11

ther by intelligence nor by a specific sense of beauty, but through the usual senses - that is, all the senses - and not only sight and hearing.

Alexander Gottlieb Baumgarten (1714–1762) published in 1750 a work in Latin entitled *Aesthetica*. It is worth recalling that this was the language in which the notion of the aesthetic was forged for the first time. According to the author, the aesthetic is the art of beautiful thought – the art of thinking in accordance with reason – and the science of sensorial recognition (*Ars pulchre cogitandi, ars analogi rationis*). The purpose of the aesthetic is to perfect sensorial recognition per se - and therefore to identify the beautiful.

In the eighteenth century, the growing tendency to subjectivize the concept of beauty culminated in the transcendental philosophy whose broad outlines were traced by Emmanuel Kant (1724–1804; fig. 13) in his *Critique of Pure Reason* (1781; fig. 12). In his treatise entitled *Critique of Judgement* he writes that there is no objective rule of taste that would define the beautiful by means of concepts: "Beauty is what is represented without a concept as an object of universal satisfaction"[1]. Since no precise concept can be adduced to determine what a beautiful appearance is, imagination and intelligence are given free rein, generating a feeling of joy which accompanies the representation of the beautiful. That is why any form of constraint is detrimental to beauty.

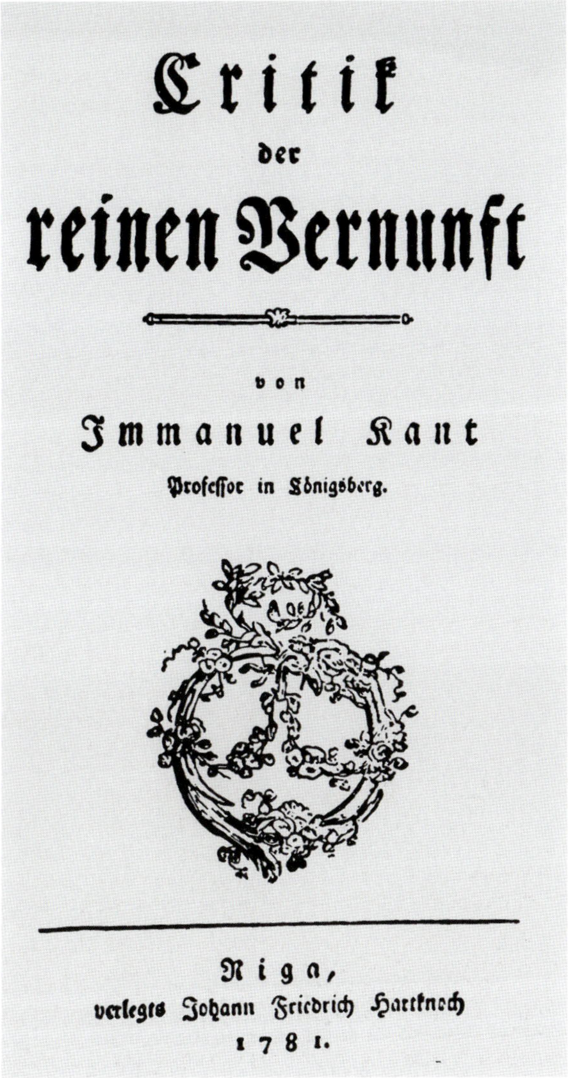

Critik
der
reinen Vernunft

von
Immanuel Kant
Professor in Königsberg.

Riga,
verlegts Johann Friedrich Hartknoch
1781.

12

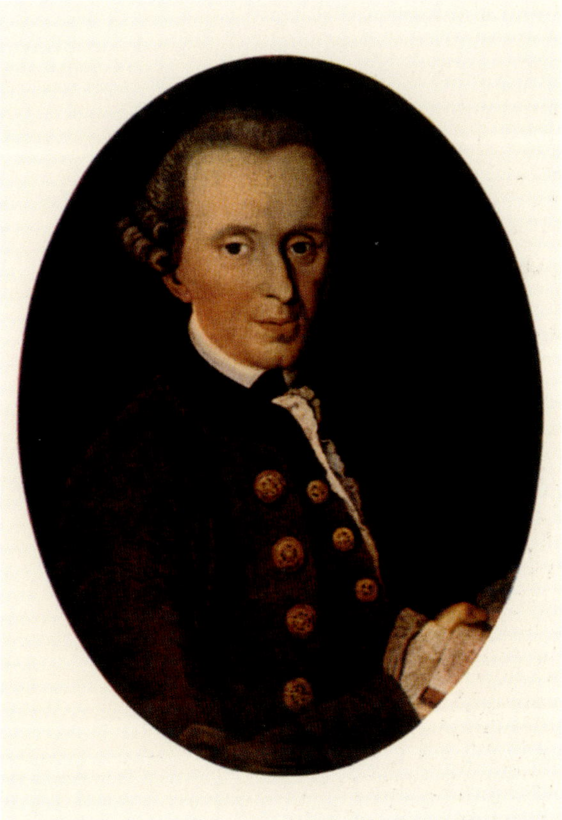

13

8 Marsilio Ficino by Andrea Ferrucci, Florence Cathedral

9 Francis Hutcheson, Hunterian Gallery, University of Glasgow

10 George Berkeley, National Portrait Gallery, London

11 Edmund Burke, unfinished portrait, private collection, in: The Great Melody, Sinclair-Stevenson, London, 1992

12 Immanuel Kant, «Kritik der reinen Vernunft», 1781, cover page, in: La saggezza dell'occidente, Longanesi, Milan, 1961

13 Immanuel Kant, in: La saggezza dell'occidente, Longanesi, Milan, 1961

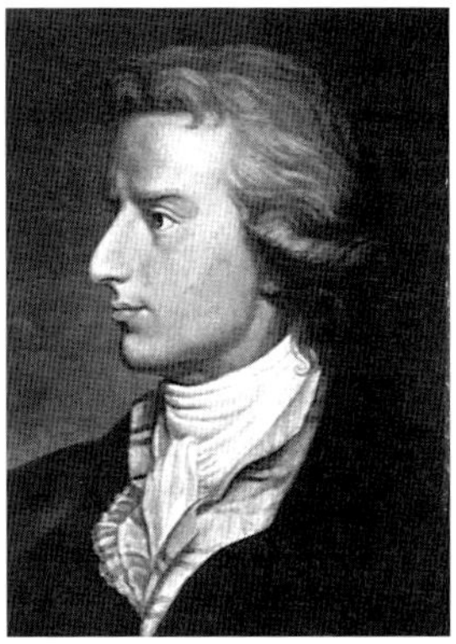

14a

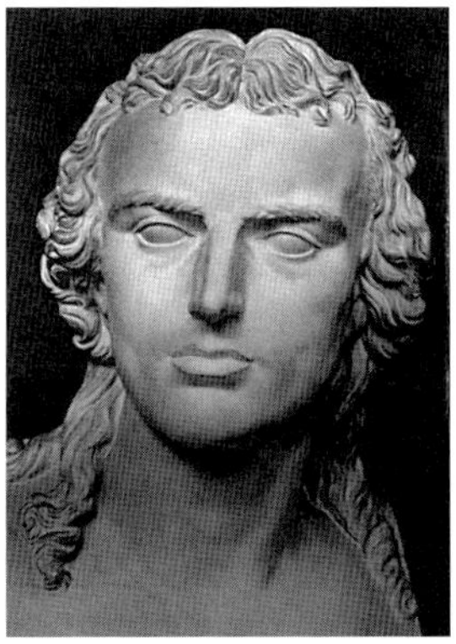

14b

In Friedrich Schiller (1759–1805; fig. 14a,b), the theory of beauty is underlaid by the desire to bring closer together the abstract and ethical dimensions of the Kantian concept of duty on the one hand, and the sensitive nature of the human being on the other. Schiller planned to lay the foundations of these principles in the form of a dialogue entitled *Kallias oder über die Schönheit*, which was to be published in 1793. The work was never written, but an outline of it can be found in a letter written to Gottfried Körner between January and February of the same year.

While for Schiller freedom was a precondition for beauty, Friedrich Nietzsche (1844–1900; fig. 15) held that nothing of what we describe as beautiful is "beautiful per se". All the beauty in the world is a reflection of our own general and individual nature, or more precisely of our instinct for self-preservation on the one hand, and of our own sense of power on the other. In principle, anything that does not conflict with our self-preservation instinct and that appeals to our sense of power is beautiful. Everything has its own beauty because the creative life force manifests itself in all things. According to Nietzsche, the fact that an object is considered to be beautiful does not reveal anything about the object, because beauty is merely a self-image, a function of its power. In his essay entitled *The Twilight of the Idols*, he writes that the beauty of a race or a family is the result of the accumulated work of generations. "It is of decisive importance for the destiny of a people and of humanity that culture begins in the right place (...): the right place is the body, physical appearance, the way of life, physiology; the rest follows from that... That is why the Greeks remain always the primary cultural event in history. They knew, and they did, what was needed; Christianity, which despised the body, has been, up to the present, the greatest misfortune of humanity."[2]

In his remarkable book entitled *Breviario di Estetica* (fig. 16), the Italian philosopher Benedetto Croce (1866–1952; fig. 17) draws some readily understandable conclusions on the theory of

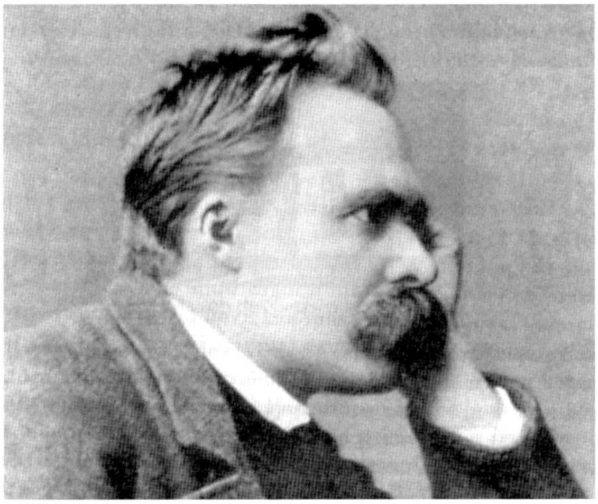

15

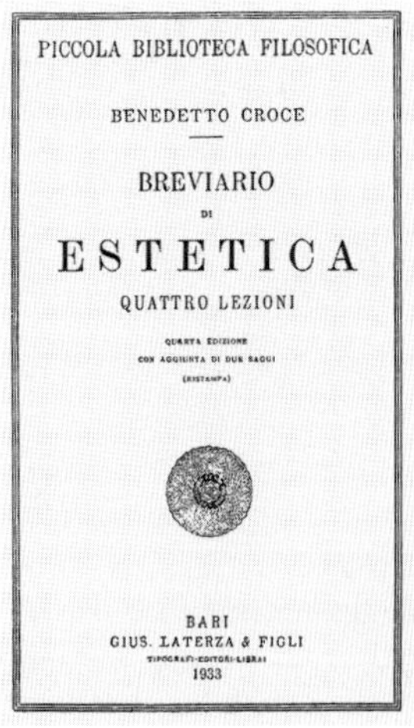

PICCOLA BIBLIOTECA FILOSOFICA

BENEDETTO CROCE

BREVIARIO

DI

ESTETICA

QUATTRO LEZIONI

BARI

GIUS. LATERZA & FIGLI

1933

16

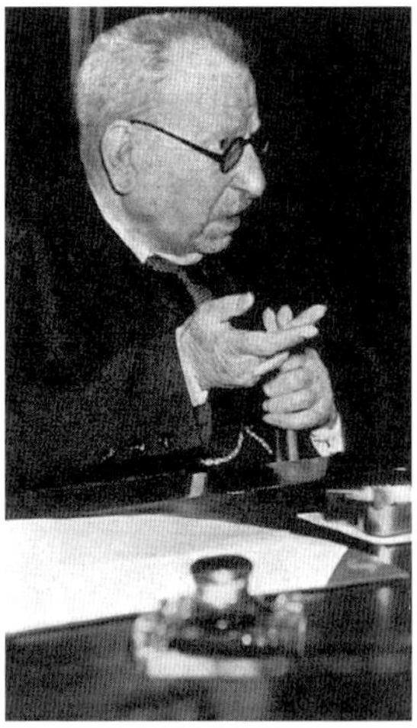

17

beauty. Beauty would have nothing to do with the physical nature of the object. Thus, the same object may or may not have a certain beauty, depending on the perspective adopted. Croce describes the results of a survey to determine the most beautiful format of an envelope. The participants' arguments tend to re-contextualize the use of the object when they explain their preferences (more elongated formats for official business, small envelopes for love letters, etc.). In essence, in Croce's view, beauty would ultimately be nothing other than the expression of the observer's perception. The object is not beautiful in itself; beauty reflects the impact of the object on the observer's mental state. With that, the concept of the beautiful definitively lost all significance and thus the 20th century aesthetic theory has largely given up using it.

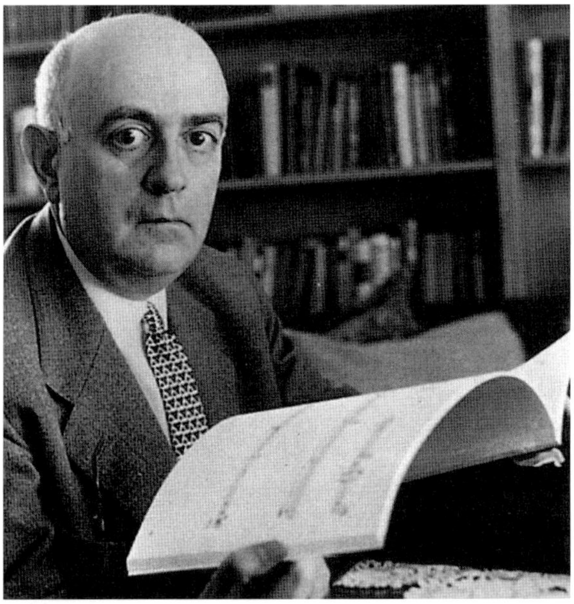

18

It was not until the aesthetic theory of Theodor W. Adorno (1903–1969; fig. 18) that the concept of the beautiful, particularly of natural beauty, became the subject of a new debate. Because it is impossible to state from the outset a criterion for what is beautiful, everything that is natural can simply become beautiful – "glowing from within". It is precisely from this fundamental uncertainty and indefiniteness of natural beauty that its essence and genuine value are distilled.

History, constantly vexed by the problem of the beautiful, has witnessed the multiple attempts to define it, increasingly over the years. It has preoccupied philosophers until today, and a constant stream of answers has been forthcoming, often partial and strongly differing.

14a Friedrich Schiller, pastel drawn by Gerhard von Kügelgen three years after the death of Schiller on the basis of existing sketches, in: Schiller, Kindler, Munich, 1958
14b Friedrich Schiller, bust by his sculptor friend Johann Heinrich Dannecker. Schiller wrote about this sculpture: "My bust has become a genuine masterpiece of astonishing authenticity...", in: Schiller, Kindler, Munich, 1958
15 Friedrich Nietzsche, 1882, the year in which he met Lou Andreas-Salom, in: Nietzsche, Pardes, Puiseaux, 2002
16 Benedetto Croce, Breviario di Estetica, 1933, cover page, in: La saggezza dell'occidente, Longanesi, Milan, 1961
17 Benedetto Croce, 1913, Rice Institute, Houston, Texas, in: La saggezza dell'occidente, Longanesi, Milan, 1961
18 Theodor W. Adorno, in: le livre des philosophes, Gallimard, Paris, 1998

[1] *Immanuel Kant, Kritik der Urteilskraft, Werkausgabe vol. 10, ed. by W. Weischedel, Suhrkamp, Frankfurt a. M., 1974, p. 124, § 6*
[2] *Friedrich Nietzsche, Götzen-Dämmerung, Streifzüge eines Unzeitgemässen, in: works in 3 vols., ed. by Karl Schlechta, vol. 2, Hanser, Munich, 1955, p. 1023*

Ideals of Beauty and Facial Proportions

Generations of artists have analysed the proportions of the human face in an attempt to define in units of measurement the criteria required for a face that is as beautiful as it is harmonious. But the first essays handed down to us on rational concepts of beauty based on proportions originate not from artists but from Greek philosophers.

The Classical Greek and Renaissance Ideals of Beauty

Pythagoras (580-497or 476 BC) and his followers reached a definition of beauty that was to become the norm all over Greece. The Pythagoreans had concerned themselves since the 6th century BC with cosmology, natural sciences and in particular with mathematics and aesthetics. They took the view that everything which is - and therefore also the properties of harmony - is determined by numbers and proportion. They attempted to find laws in the numbers to give an ordered framework to reality. For them, the world became the *kosmos*, a rationally comprehensible order. But this means nothing other than that the world is beautiful, because the Greek word *kalos* is generally understood as beauty. For the Pythagoreans, beauty was nothing other than order in the sense of an objective characteristic of reality which manifested itself in form as *harmonia* (order and proportion) and as *symmetria* (good proportion corresponding to

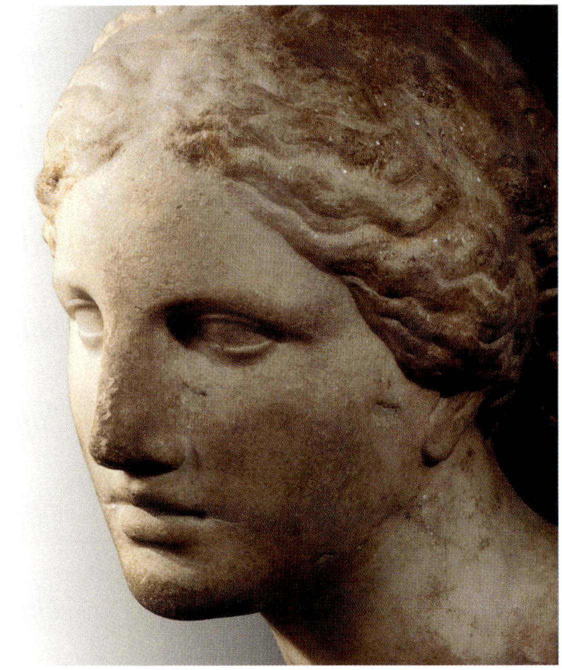

1

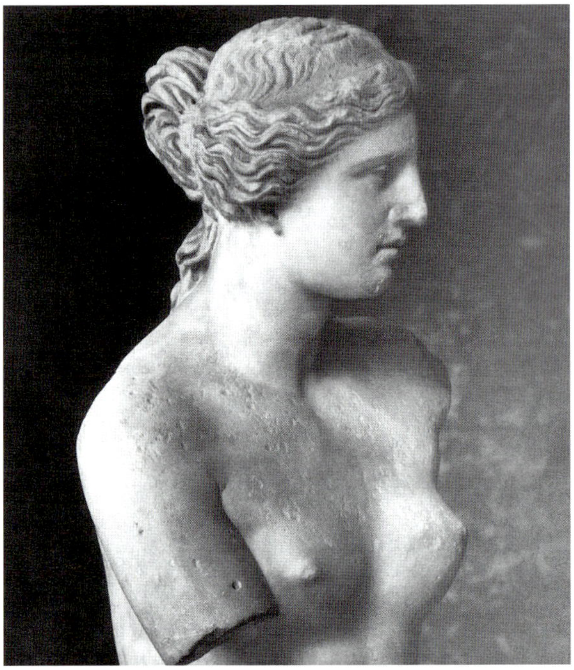

2

the right measure). Measure and proportion became the basis for planning and action in the various spheres of art - at first in music and architecture and later in painting and in sculpture.

Aristotle (384–322 BC), who followed in the footsteps of his master Plato by studying exact sciences – namely arithmetic, geometry, astronomy and harmonics – discussed the Pythagoreans' theories and mathematical insights in his writings. In keeping with the Pythagorean tradition, the main characteristics of beauty were precision, symmetry and coordination – as demonstrated in the mathematical sciences – and they were therefore also determining for the aesthetics of the human face.

Many Greek sculptors – Polycletus (480–420 BC) and Praxiteles (390–325 BC) for example – expressed in their works the perfect beauty of the human form, based on ideal proportions. The Aphrodite by Praxiteles (fig. 1), the Venus de Milo (fig. 2) and many other sculptures (figs. 3–5) embody the aesthetic ideal of ancient Greece. Praxiteles's Aphrodite is thought to have been sculpted between 350 and 330 BC.. It is said that Praxiteles used Phryne, his mistress, as a model for this sculpture depicting the goddess of love and embodiment of beauty. Phryne was a very famous woman, as well known for her beauty as for her aptitude to use her physical charm to manipulate the rich Athenians and the important politicians. She seems to have been the courtesan of many politicians. Legend has it that she once was brought to trial because of the blasphemous act of disrobing and walking naked into the sea before a crowd of people attending the festivities of Poseidon. In court, she revealed her bare bosom before the judges, arguing that she was too beautiful to commit a crime. Subsequently, she was judged not guilty. Phryne also used her beauty to benefit her native country of Greece. When the walls of Thebes were destroyed by Alexander the Great in 335 B.C., she collected the money for their restoration.

The Venus de Milo is so well known that it embodies its own myth of beauty. It was discovered in 1820 on the island of Melos and is thought to have been sculpted about 150 BC by a little-known artist from Antioch named Alexandros.

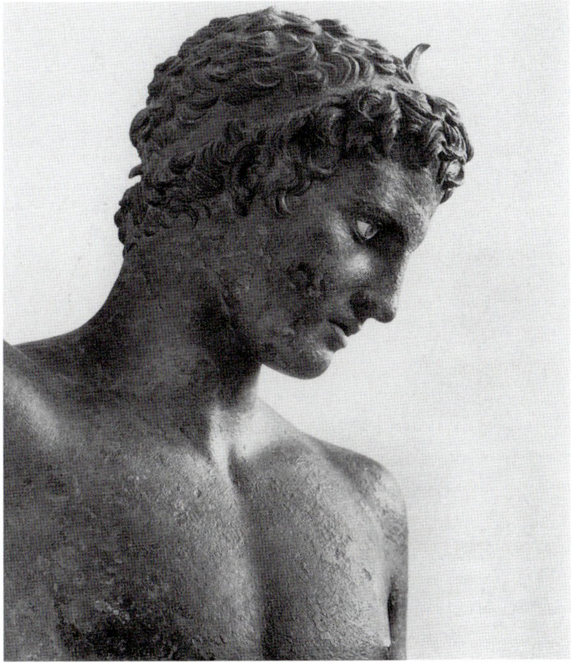

3

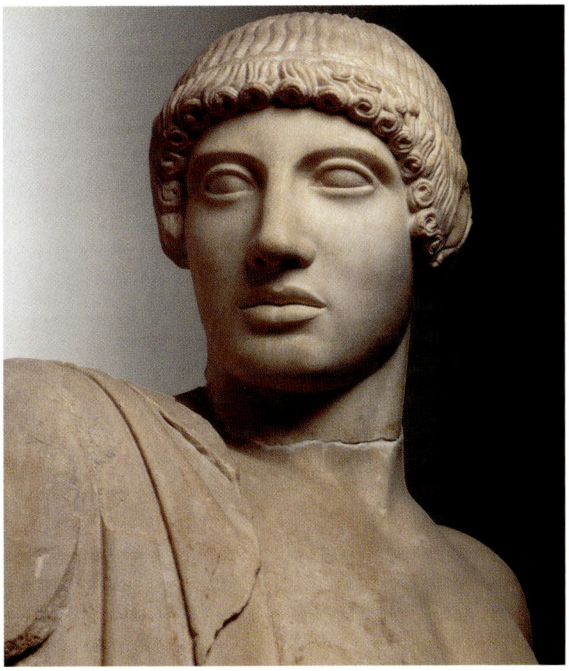

4

1 Aphrodite by Praxiteles (350–330 BC), The Louvre, Paris

2 Venus de Milo, The Louvre, Paris

3 Ephebe of Marathon (340–330 BC), bronze, National Museum, Athens

4 Head of Apollo, 1st century BC, Temple of Zeus, Archaeological Museum, Olympia

During the Renaissance all great artists reappraised the works of Antiquity and the ideals of beauty inherent in them. This harking back, as expressed in the Renaissance works, reflects the classical ideals of beauty. Implementation of the theory which holds that beauty is based on the harmony of its forms attained a high degree of perfection in the Renaissance. The heritage of Antiquity was seen in a new light, particularly by the Florentine prince Cosimo de Medici and the philosopher of whom he was the patron, Marsilio Ficino (1438–1499 AD).

The world appeared to be a great work of art which, through its beauty, is blessed with the fullness of the divine. But bodies first have to be rendered reflective of beauty through order, proportion and shaping *(ordo, modus, species)*. This beauty, which in turn results from the balanced proportions of its parts, appears to be all the more "radiant" the closer it approaches beauty. During the Renaissance it thus attained a high symbolic value. The Renaissance artist was both an imitator of nature and a creator of a new reality (figs. 17–23).

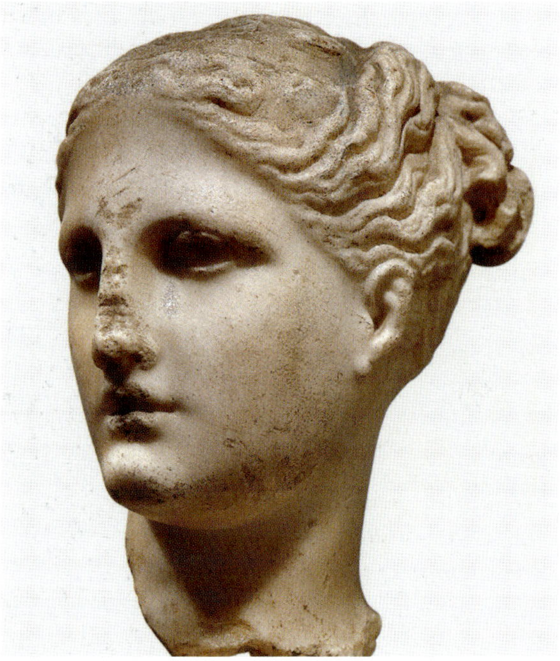

5

In his essay *Of Beauty*, the philosopher Francis Bacon (1561–1626; fig. 16) reminds us that "virtue is like a rich stone, best plain set; and surely virtue is best in a body that is comely, though not of delicate features; and that hath rather dignity of presence than beauty of aspect. Neither is it almost seen, that very beautiful persons are otherwise of great virtue; as if Nature were rather busy not to err, than in labour to produce excellency."[1] But this rule allows for some exceptions, Bacon tells us: "Augustus Cæsar, Titus Vespasianus, Philip le Bel of France, Edward the Fourth of England, Alcibiades of Athens and Ismael the Sophy of Persia were all high and great spirits and yet the most beautiful men of their times. In beauty, that of favour is more than

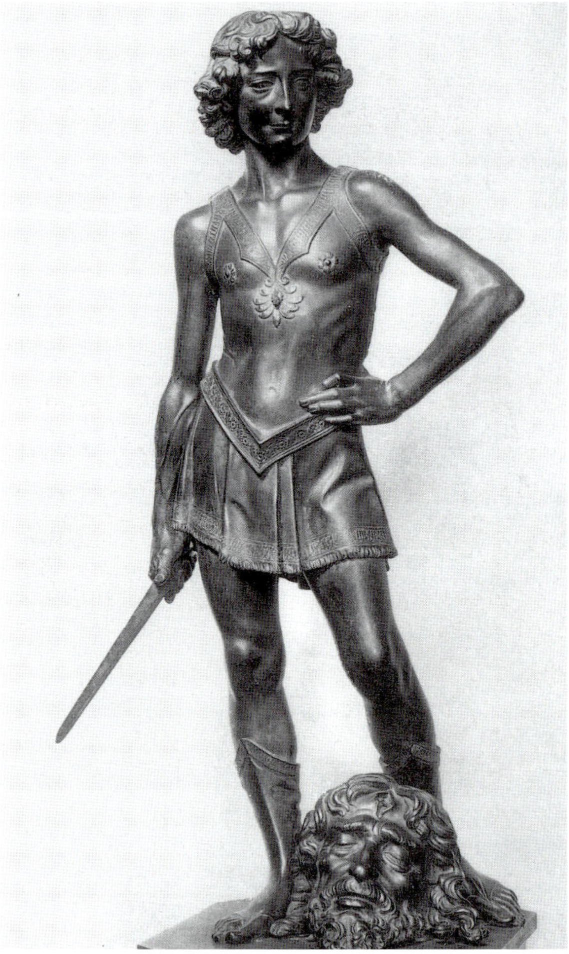

6a

that of colour; and that of decent and gracious motion, more than that of favour. That is the best part of beauty, which a picture cannot express."[1] Bacon notes that there are faces which, when examined part by part, do not look very beautiful; but when perceived as a whole these parts yield up beauty.

Studies on Facial Proportions by Leonardo da Vinci and Albrecht Dürer

The two leading Renaissance artists Leonardo da Vinci and Albrecht Dürer, more than anyone else, analysed the proportions of the human body and face in the quest for a fundamental and generally valid definition of beauty. They recorded their insights in their many sketches and scientific treatises.

Leonardo da Vinci (1452–1519), depicted here in the bronze sculpture by his master Andrea del Verrocchio and in the painting by Francesco Botticini as a youth (figs. 6a,b, 7), wrote numerous documents in which he examined in detail aesthetic theories and theories of the proportions of the human body. He was impressed by, among other things, the theories of the Roman architect Markus Vitruvius Pollio (70–25 BC). Influenced by Vitruvius's portrayal of a man standing up with outstretched arms within a square, Leonardo da Vinci created his own version of the proportions of the person standing with his legs apart and arms stretched upwards, but in a circle: "If you spread your legs sufficiently for your height to be reduced by one fourteenth, and if you open and raise your arms so that the middle fingers touch the line originating at the top of your head, your navel will be half way between the ends of your outstretched limbs; and the space between your legs will form an equilateral triangle. The span of a man's outstretched arms is equal to his height"[2] (fig. 9).

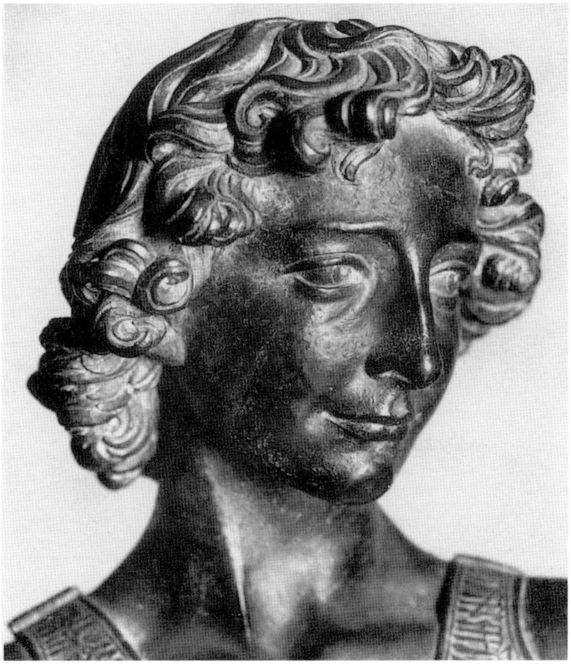

6b

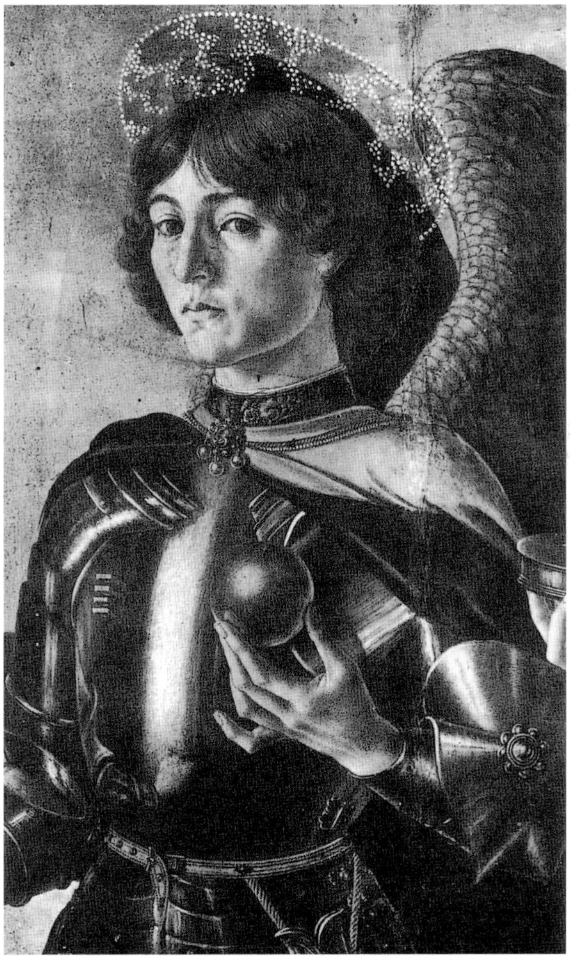

7

5 Head of a woman, 1st century BC, National Archaeological Museum, Taranto

6a David by Andrea del Verrocchio, National Museum of Bargello, Florence. Bronze executed in Verrocchio's atelier where Leonardo da Vinci worked. It is presumed that the 20 year-old Leonardo posed as the model for this statue

6b David, detail of the face, by Andrea del Verrocchio, National Museum of Bargello, Florence.

7 Francesco Botticini, Archangel Michael, with the features of Leonardo da Vinci, Uffizi Gallery, Florence

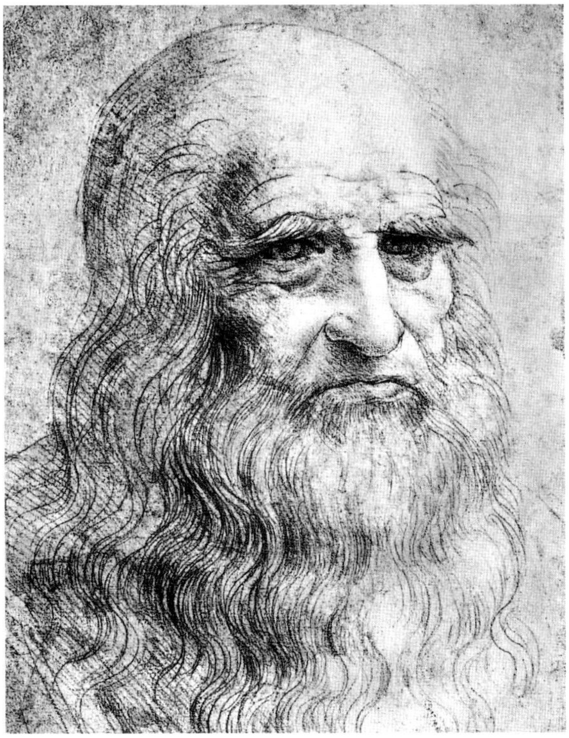

8

In his quest to gain scientific insights, Leonardo da Vinci investigated the proportions of a human face from a wide range of angles. He used the well-known basic division of the face into three equal parts and sub-divided it with additional horizontal, vertical and oblique coordinates. This analysis is explained in his two famous sketches (figs. 10, 11). Leonardo presumably used himself as a model, as these faces are very similar to his only self-portrait, which is thought to have been painted at the age of 62 (fig. 8). Here are just some of his observations on the proportions of the human face: "The elements that are located between the chin and the nose, between the latter and the eyebrows, and between the latter and the hairline each measure as much as the ear and each represents one third of the face (...). The lines from the eyebrow to the junction of the lip with the chin, and from there to the (posterior) edge of the jaw, and from there to the upper edge of the ear, near the temple, form a perfect square, the side of which measures half the head"[2] (fig. 10). "The face forms a square, the

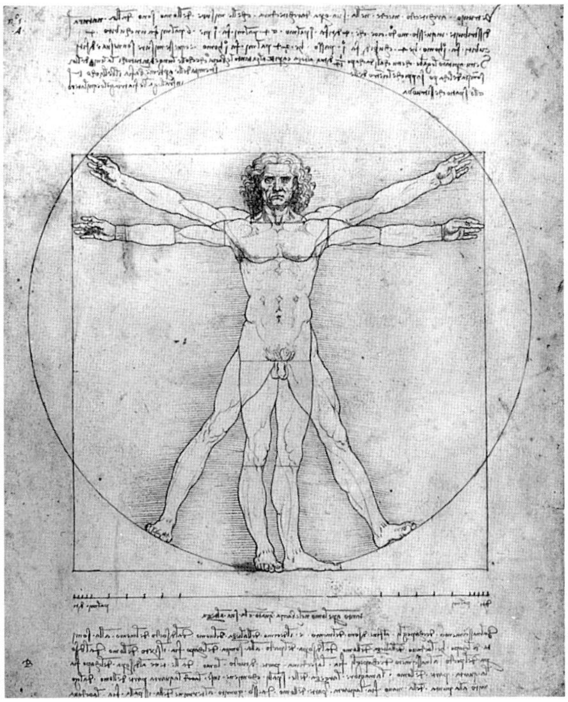

9

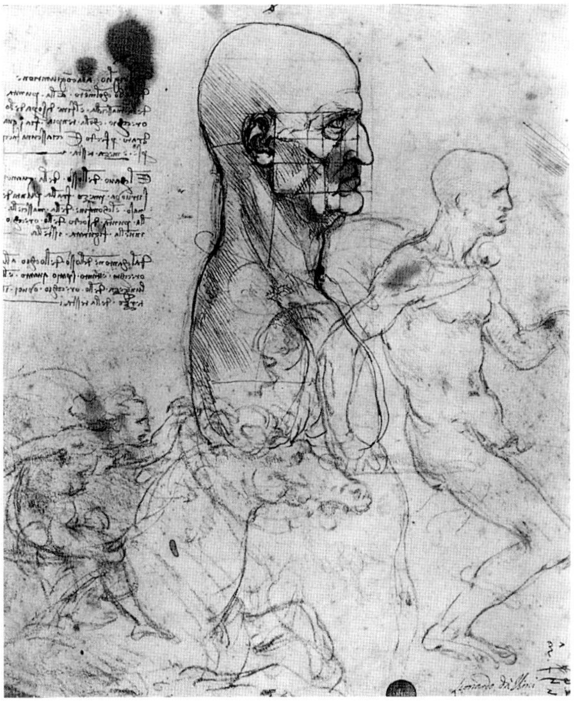

10

width of which goes from one end of the eye to the other, and the height goes from the top of the nose to the lower edge of the lower lip"[2] (fig. 11). "The cavity beneath the cheekbones is located mid-way between the tip of the nose and the end of the jawbone"[2] (fig. 10). "The distance between the eyes is equal to the width of one eye"[2] (fig. 11). "The distance between the two pupils is equal to one third of the face"[2] (fig. 11). "From the outer edge of the orbita to the ear the distance is equal to the length of the ear, in other words, one third of the head"[2] (fig. 10). And with regard to the ratio between face and body, he noted: "From the hairline to the base of the chin, there is one tenth of a man's height; from the base of the chin to the top of the head, one eighth of a man's height."[2]

Leonardo's observations on facial proportions can be summarized with one of his well-known maxims: that every part of the whole has to be in proportion to the whole. But Leonardo subordinated his theories of proportions and the harmony of the human face to the human being's inner radiance or suprasensuous beauty. It is on this conviction that his famous advice to future artists is based: "A good painter must reveal two main things: the image of man and the essence of his mind."[2] This maxim is put into practice in many of the master's inspired portraits, in which the human being's inner and outer beauty become one.

Like Leonardo da Vinci, Albrecht Dürer (1471–1528; fig. 15), studied the proportions of the human body and face intensively and he set out his manifold insights in four richly-illustrated books entitled *Proportions of the Human Body*. In the illustration reproduced here of a male face in profile, Dürer was experimenting with a square which he subdivided with a network of coordinates: seven horizontal and five vertical equally-spaced coordinates (fig. 13a,b). Two of them are located in the front part of the head and encompass the eye, while three of them are in the rear part of the head, the front two of which delimiting the front and rear edge of the ear. An additional vertical

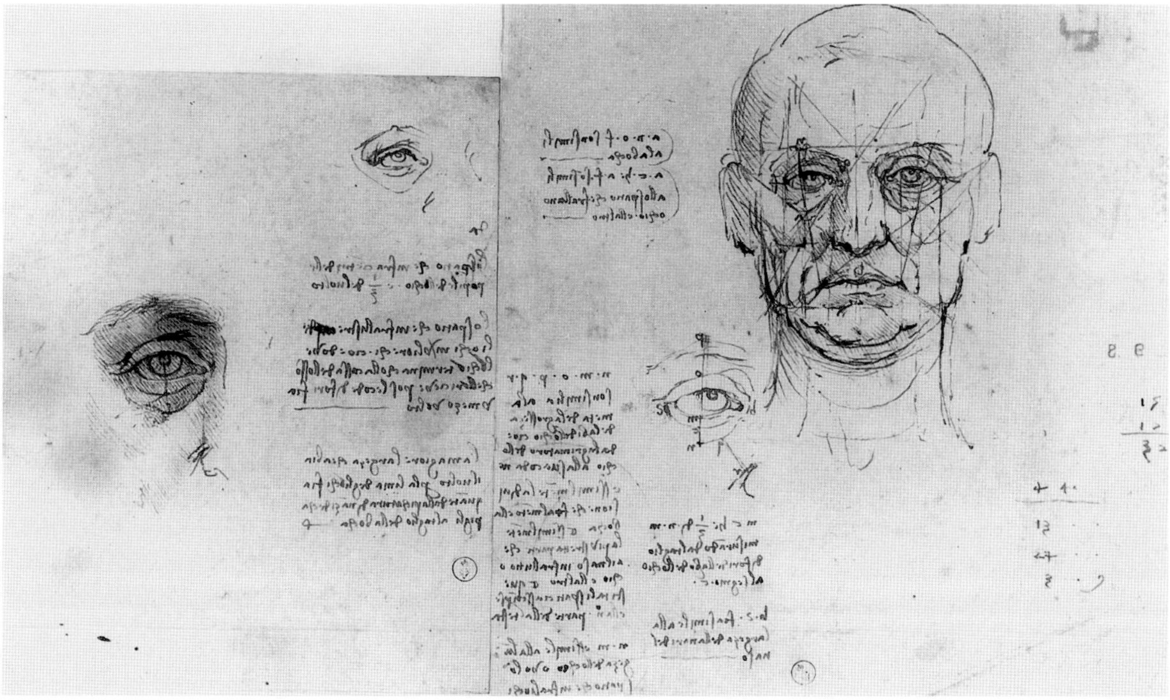

11

8 Self-portrait of Leonardo da Vinci, Royal Library, Turin

9 Leonardo da Vinci, the proportions of the human body, Gallerie dell'Accademia, Venice

10 Leonardo da Vinci, study of the proportions of the face, Gallerie dell'Accademia, Venice

11 Leonardo da Vinci, studies of the proportions of the face and the eyes, Royal Library, Turin

line divides the head into two equal parts (fig. 13a,b). In this sketch Dürer places the highest point of the cranium (A) over the mastoid (B) and the broadest point on the rear side of the cranium (C) at the level of the glabella of the frontal bone (D). Interestingly enough, Dürer modified line (E) in his sketch so that the neck line (F) runs vertically onto the newly-drawn line (E) and onto line (G), which extends along the lower part of the face. The line J - G that he drew corresponds to the "aesthetic line" reproduced in some aesthetic facial surgery textbooks, with which the position of the lips is determined in relation to the nose and chin region.

Dürer's horizontal division of the face follows the conventional division into three equal parts between the frontal hairline (H), eyebrow (J), base of the nose (K) and chin (L). However, the distance from the hairline (H) to the top of the head (I) is greater than usual and in this case is as large as each one third of the face (H–J, J–K, K–L). With these three horizontal lines (H, J, K) Dürer divides the head into four equally-sized parts. The upper part of the eyebrow (J) and the base of the nose (K) coincide with the upper and lower edge of the ear. In his third and fourth books, Albrecht Dürer depicted the proportions of a wide range of different human faces. The third book also contains some principles for portraying a generally valid, ideal harmony of the human face. The artist notes that there is not a single human being in the world who combines all the elements of beauty in his or her person, as the individual could always

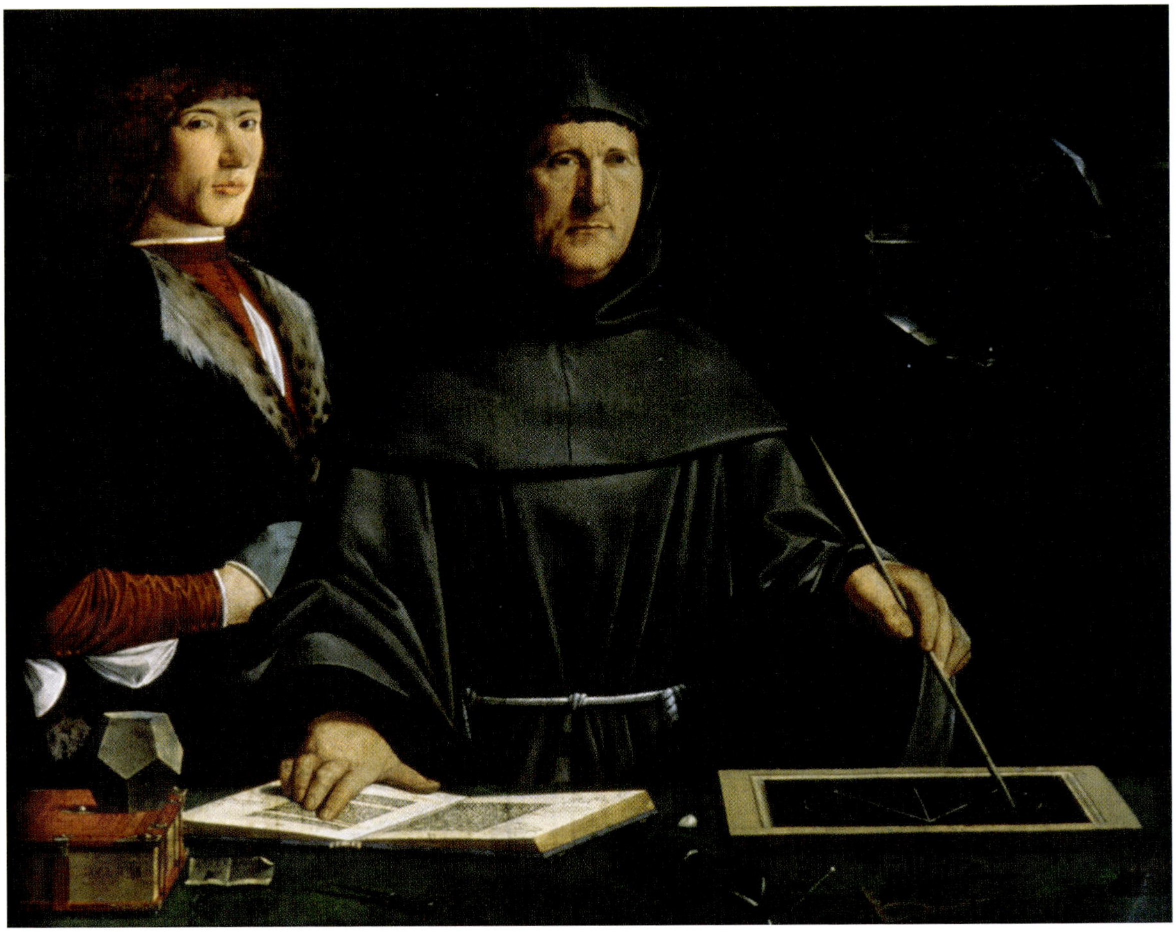

12

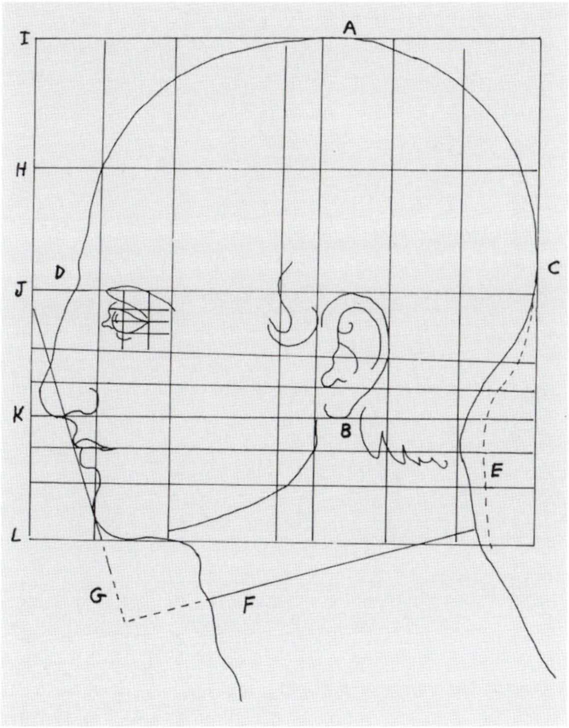

13a

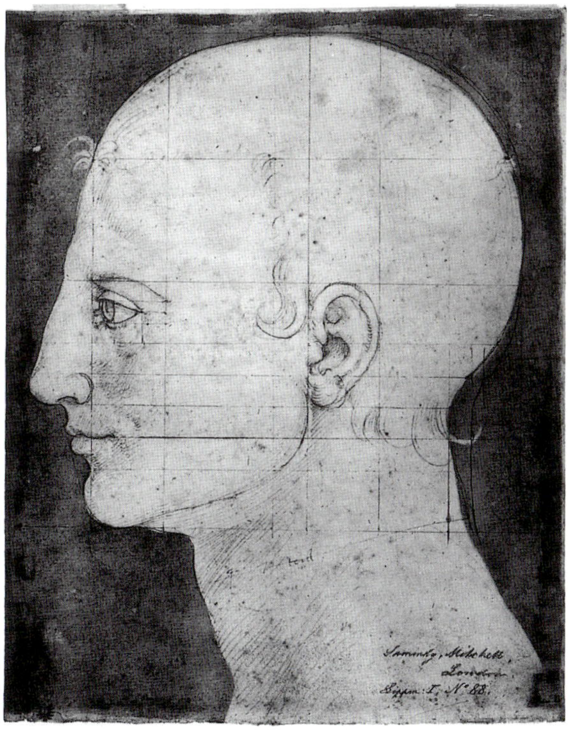

13b

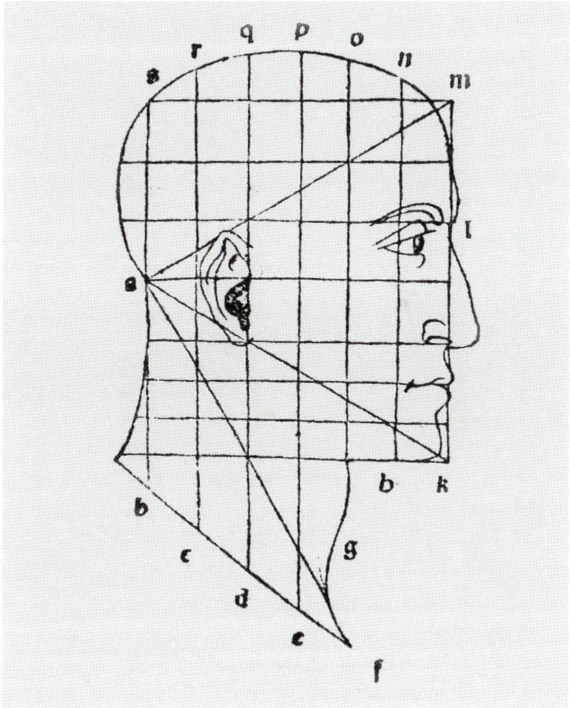

14

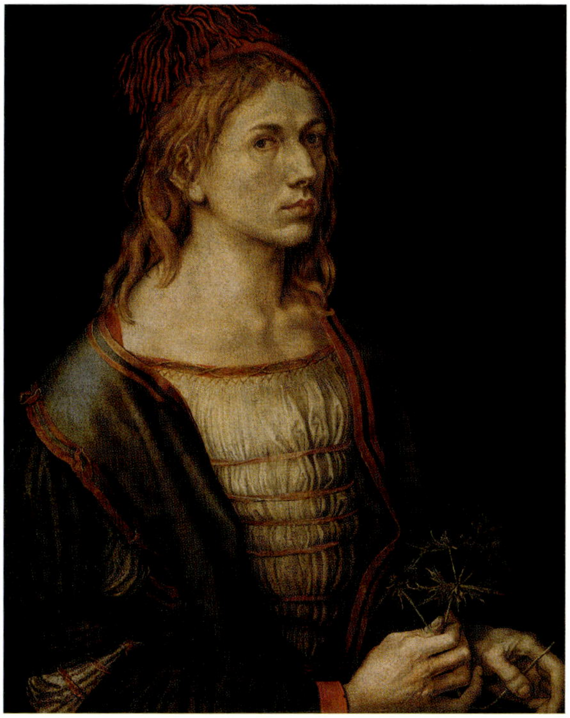

15

12 Jacopo de Barbari, Friar Luca Pacioli, National Museum of Capodimonte, Naples
13a Albrecht Dürer, construction of the head in profile, Pierpont Morgan Library, New York
13b Schematic drawing of the illustration 13a, in: Anatomy Lessons from the Great Masters, Robert Beverly Hale, Terence Coyle, Watson-Guptill Publ., New York, 1977
14 Presumed portrait by Leonardo da Vinci in "Divina proportione" by Friar Luca Pacioli, in: Leonardo da Vinci, vol. 1, Istituto Geografico de Agostini, Novara, 1956
15 Albrecht Dürer, self-portrait, 1493, The Louvre, Paris

be even more beautiful. Nor is there a single person, he continues, who can define human beauty. Our judgment of human beauty is so full of doubt, in Dürer's view, that when we meet two very graceful and beautiful people we cannot say which is the more beautiful, although the two persons would not resemble one another in any part of their body, neither in their proportions nor in their character. It can happen that one studies two or three hundred human faces to find two or three beautiful elements. In general, the "average", "rational" features, that is, those that are not exaggerated, are the better ones and are more graceful. Another well-known phenomenon, Dürer continued, is our inclination to regard also as beautiful a face that everyone else considers to be beautiful. Dürer rejects this conventional conception of beauty. In order to portray a beautiful face, it has to be given excellent proportions. For this purpose measurements need to be carried out on many persons who are considered beautiful. Equally great attention should be paid to the whole face and to its individual parts – that is,

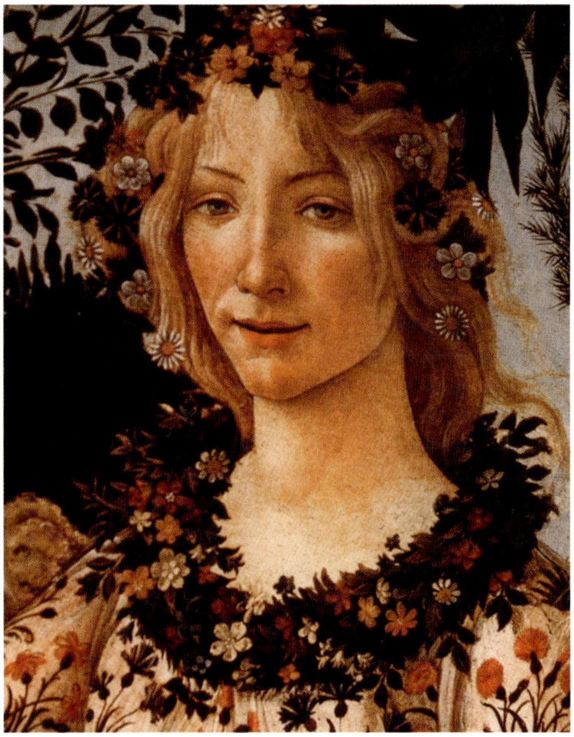

17

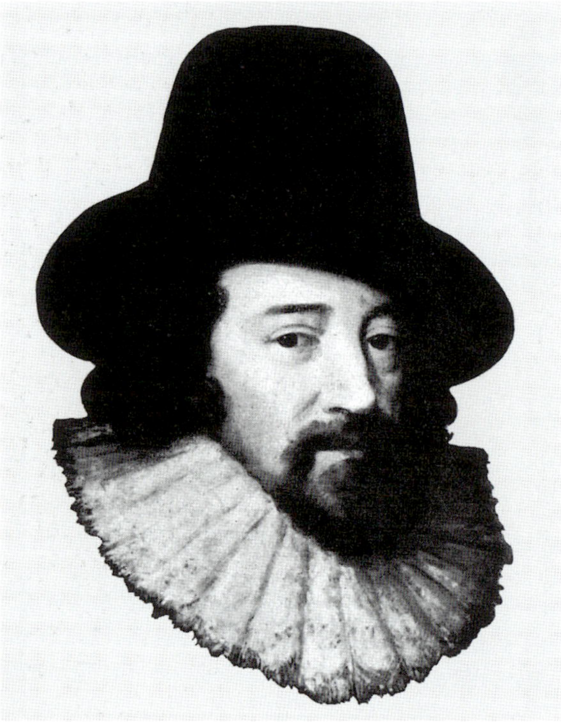

16

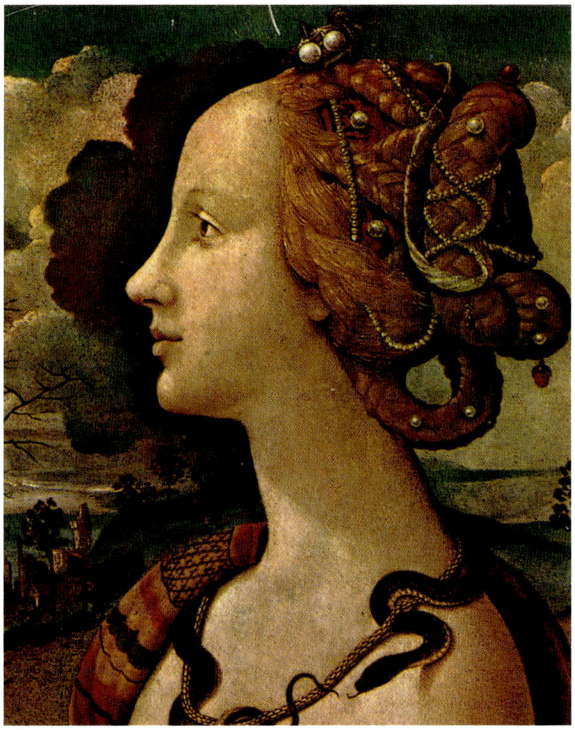

18

forehead, nose, eyes and mouth – without neglecting the slightest details. "You can't prevent a person from making a beautiful impression. For there's not a person on this earth who is beautiful in every respect, he would always fain be more handsome. Nor is there a single person on earth who could definitively say what the most beautiful person would look like. Nobody knows save God alone. (...) For in many things we regard as beautiful something that would not be beautiful in another person. It is not easy for us to distinguish beautiful from more beautiful (...) I know not what beauty is, although it is attached to many things!"[3]

The re-discovery of the arithmetic properties of certain numbers that ancient authors had observed triggered almost mythical rapture among the Renaissance artists. This applies in particular to the golden ratio ("proportio divina" or "sectio aurea") which was described by the famous Greek mathematician Euclid (330–270 BC) in around 300 BC and was applied in the following centuries by many sculptors and architects. In 1509 the mathematician and Franciscan friar Luca Pacioli from Borgo San Sepolcro (1445–1514; fig. 12) published his work *De Divina Proportione* in Venice. It is one of the first treatises to focus on the Golden Ratio. In this book, the scientist presents mathematical properties, aesthetic characteristics and some mystic properties of the Golden Ratio. Luca Pacioli wrote this book at the court of Lodovico Sforza, Duke of Milan, who was known as il Moro and according to friar Luca Pacioli some illustrations are supposed to have originated from Leonardo da Vinci, who at the time was also in the Duke's employ (fig. 14).

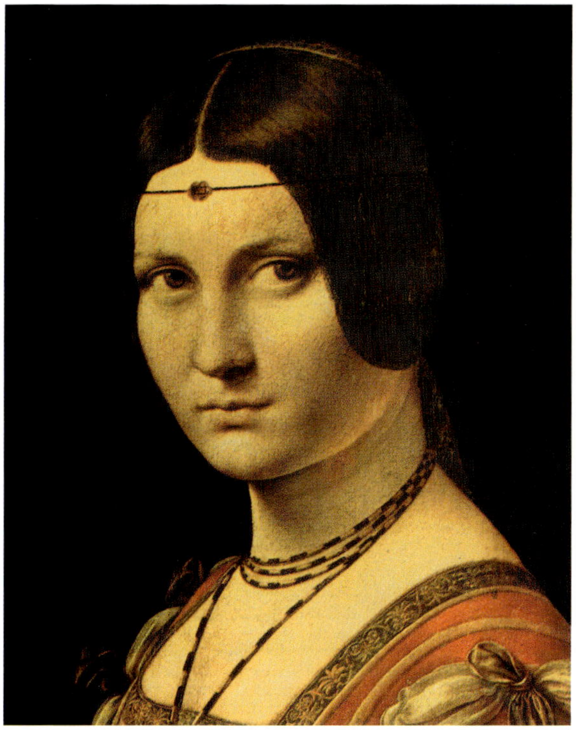

19

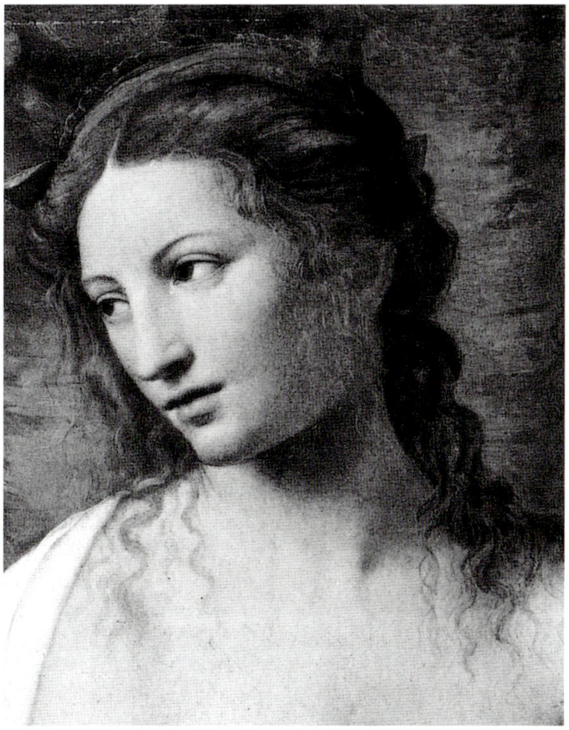

20

16 Paul van Somer, Francis Bacon, National Portrait Gallery, London

17 Sandro Botticelli, Spring, Uffizi Gallery, Florence

18 Piero di Cosimo, Simonetta Vespucci, Condé Museum, Chantilly

19 Leonardo da Vinci, La Belle Ferronnière, The Louvre, Paris

20 Bernardino Luini, Susanna, Prince Borromeo collection, Milan

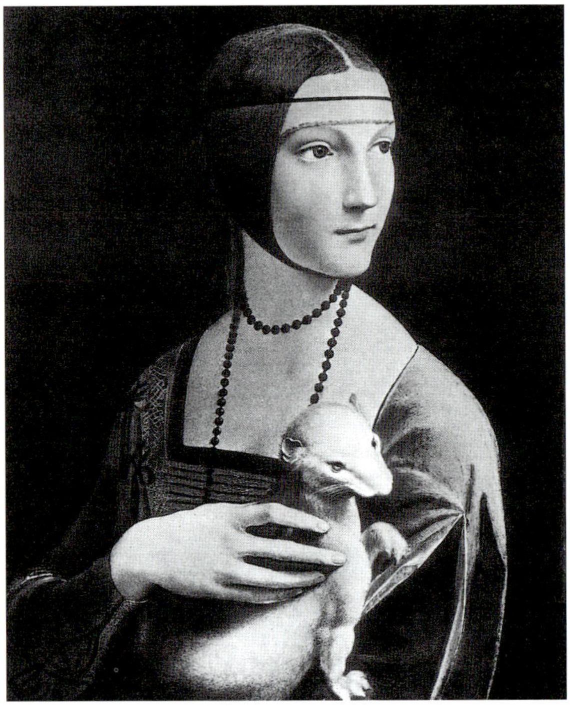

21

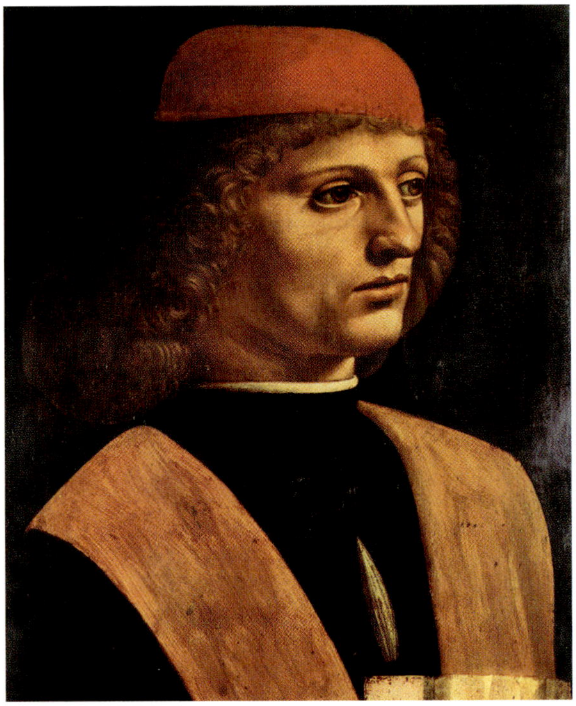

22

[1] *For this and the following quotations, see Francis Bacon, The Essays, Mount Vernon, N.Y., 1940, pp. 168-169*

[2] *For this and the following quotations of Leonardo da Vinci, see Leonardo da Vinci, "The problems of the painter", in: Sämtliche Gemälde und die Schriften zur Malerei, edited by André Chastel, Munich: Schirmer-Mosel 1990, pp. 288-293, p.305*

[3] *Albrecht Dürer, über die Proportionen des menschlichen Körpers, in: ders., Schriften und Briefe, edited by Ernst Ullmann, Leipzig: Reclam 1978, p. 127*

21 Leonardo da Vinci, Lady with an Ermine, Czartoryski Museum, Cracow
22 Leonardo da Vinci, drawing of a musician, Pinacoteca Ambrosiana, Milan

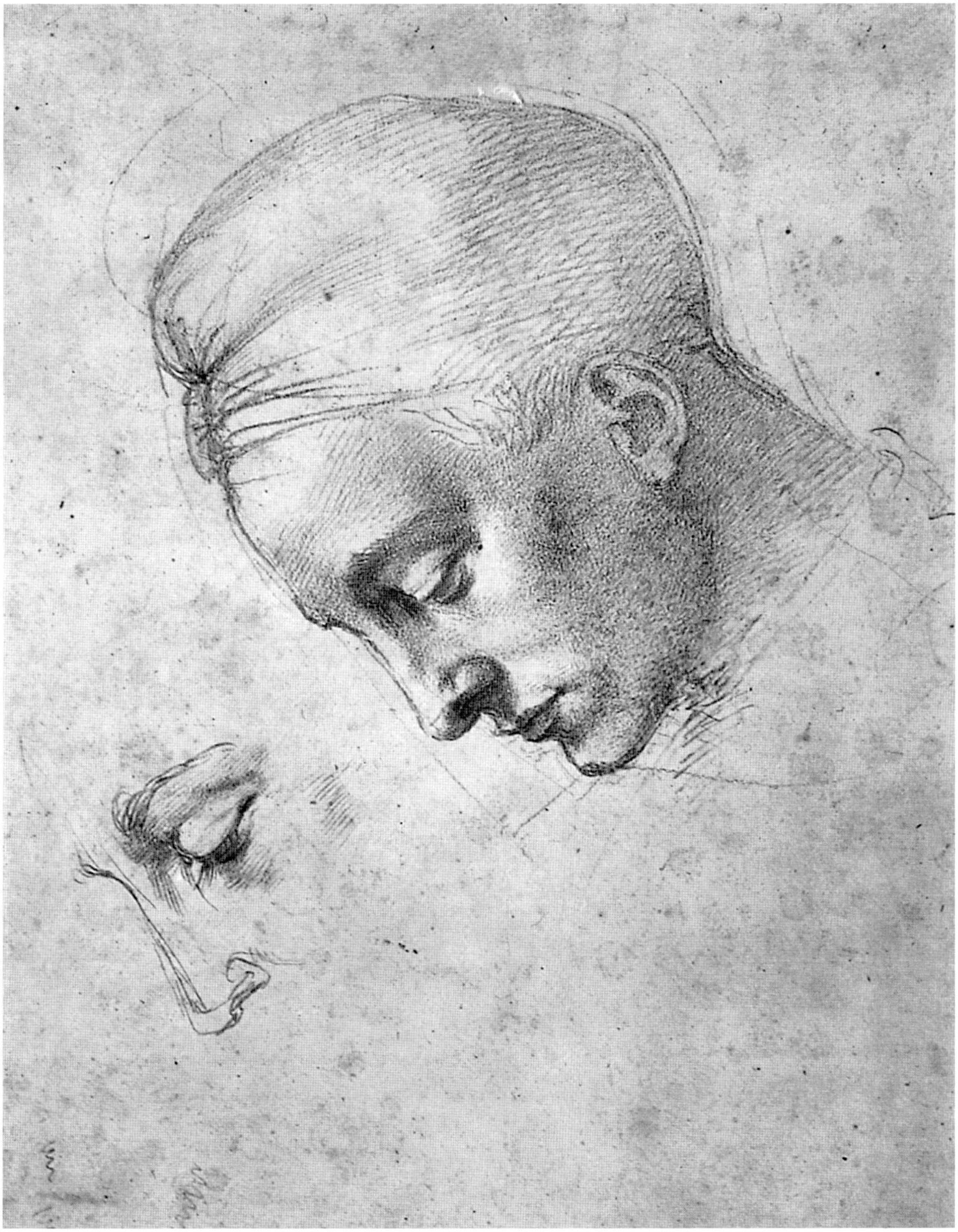

23

23 Michelangelo, study of head, Casa Buonarotti, Florence

My Own Studies of Facial Proportions

Based on the proportion studies by Leonardo da Vinci and Albrecht Dürer, I studied, using photographs, the facial proportions of more than fifty world-famous figures whom I consider to be beautiful such as Marilyn Monroe, Grace Kelly, Brigitte Bardot, Capucine, Isa Stoppi, Marlon Brando, Clark Gable and Claudia Schiffer. In doing so I observed that these faces fit – almost without exception - into a diagram of proportions which I had proposed and which was inspired by the works of Leonardo and Dürer (figs. 24, 25, 26). My basic diagram consists solely of vertical and horizontal coordinates, which are all the same distance from one another.

In the side view I depicted the head - as in Dürer's sketch - in a square with the conventional threefold horizontal division of the face by the coordinates k, l, m, but with a sevenfold vertical and sevenfold horizontal division of the head (fig. 27a). I designated the individual coordinates with small letters, in the same order in which Dürer used them in his various proportional diagrams. I also portrayed the face frontally in a square and divided it with the identical system of coordinates as in the side view (fig. 27b). The two outer vertical segments, which each correspond to one seventh of the side of the square, are located outside the face, bordering on the auricle. The face itself is divided by the six vertical coordinates a, c, d, e, f, b into five equally large vertical segments, each of which is exactly as large as each of the seven segments in the side view. In this division it can clearly be seen that the distance between the eyes corresponds to one fifth of the frontal measurement and is equivalent to the breadth of an eye or to the width of the nose in the region of its base. The part of the cranium above the upper third of the face in my drawing is one seventh of the total height of the head and is an average of the corresponding measurements in the proportional sketches by Leonardo and Dürer (figs. 13a,b, 14, 32a,b). The face is divided into two halves by a horizontal median line x and by a vertical median line y (figs. 27a,b). The horizontal

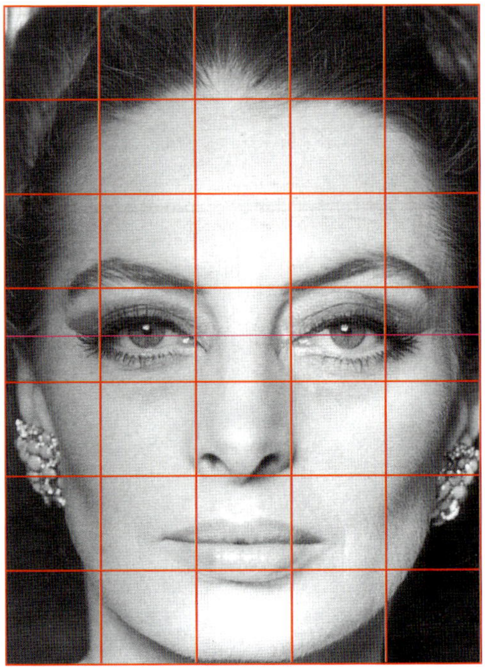

24

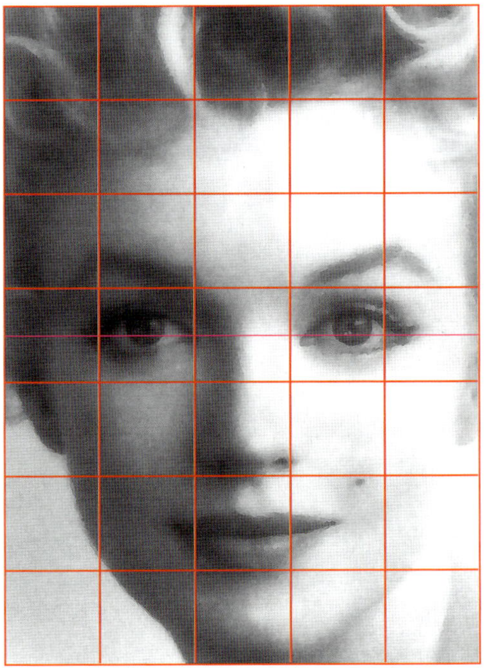

25

24 Capucine, 1968, Rome, photograph by Gian Paolo Barbieri, with diagram of proportions by Urs Victor Burki

25 Marilyn Monroe, 1956, with diagram of proportions by Urs Victor Burki. Photo: Monroe Image, © 2005 Milton H. Greene Archives, Inc. www.archivesmhg.com

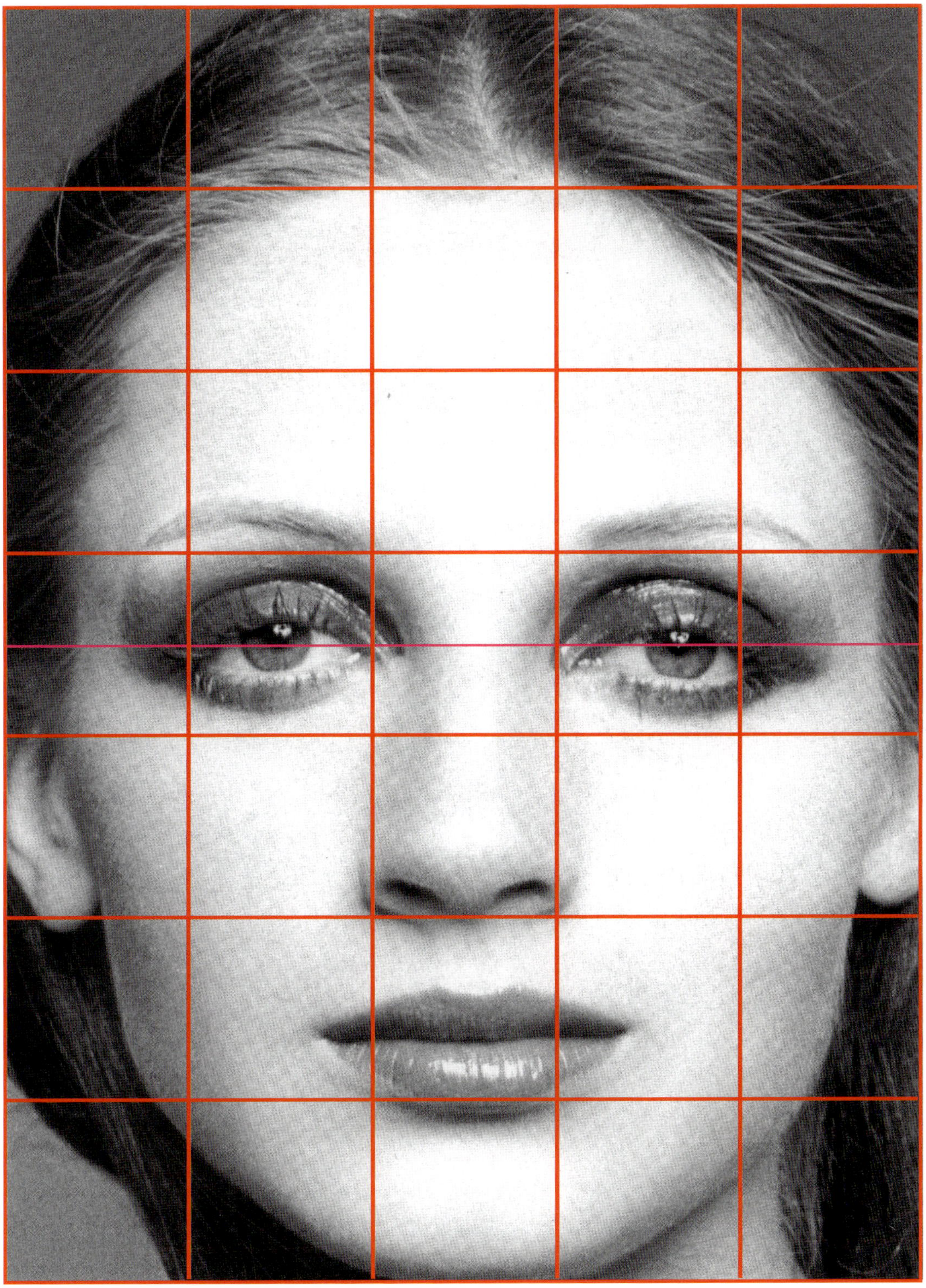

26

26 Isa Stoppi, 1965, Milan, photograph by Gian Paolo Barbieri, with diagram of proportions by Urs Victor Burki

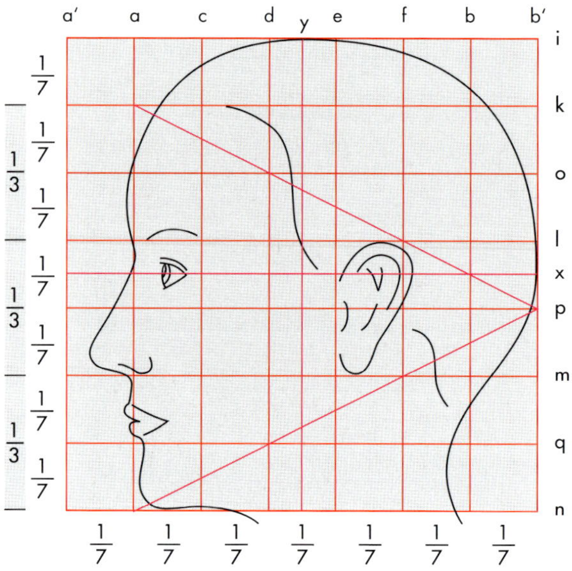

27a

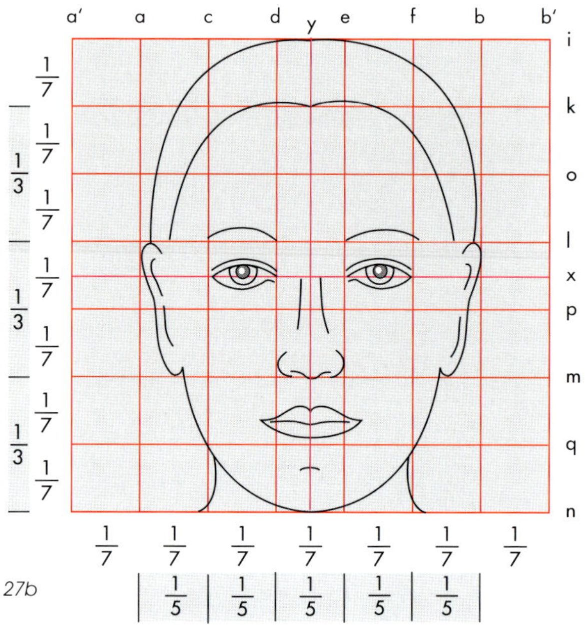

27b

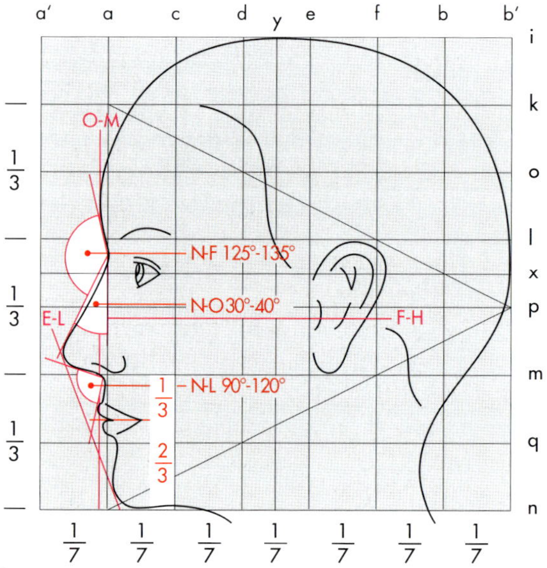

27c

meridian line is situated at the level of the outer canthi (figs. 27a,b). The widest point on the rear side of the cranium, at the occiput, in the profile view of the face is located in the region of the point of contact of line x with the side of square b' and the highest point of the cranium in the region of the point of contact of line y with the side I of the square (fig. 27a).

The length of the ear corresponds in my schema of proportions to one third of the face. The nose is slightly shorter than the middle third of the face whereas its length in the drawings of proportions by Leonardo and Dürer corresponds to one third of the face (figs. 13a,b, 14, 27a,b).

According to Leonardo's sketch, I divided the lower third of the face into one upper and two lower thirds (fig. 27c). The upper third extends from the base of the nose - or from coordinate m - to the junction between the upper and lower lip, the stomion; the lower two thirds extend from the stomion to the lowest point of the chin soft tissue, which touches coordinate n (fig. 27c). In this figure I have also drawn in the "O - meridian line" (O-M), which is named after the plastic surgeon Mario Gonzalez-Ulloa (1961) and is used in aes-

27a Basic diagram of the proportions of the face, profile, drawing by Urs Victor Burki

27b Basic diagram of the proportions of the face, front view, drawing by Urs Victor Burki

27c Basic diagram of the proportions of the face, with angle measurements, profile, drawing by Urs Victor Burki

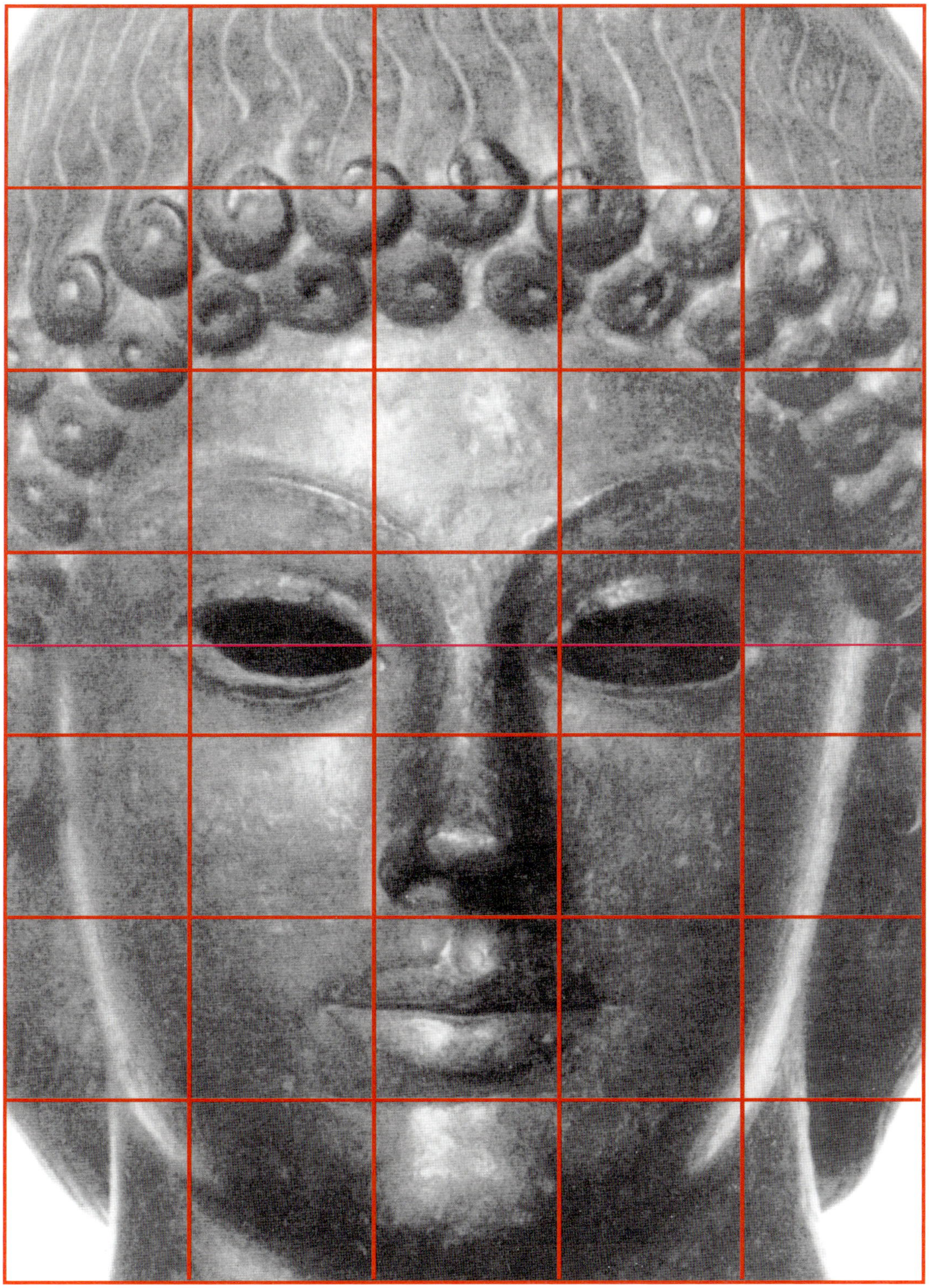

28

28 Apollo of Piombino, The Louvre, Paris, with diagram of proportions by Urs Victor Burki thetic surgery to judge the shape and position of the nose and chin. This line runs vertically along the glabella and at a right angle to the so-called "Frankfurt horizontal" line (F–H; fig. 27c). A line that is generally used to judge the lower half of the face - the aesthetic line (E–L) – is already visible in Dürer's proportional sketch (figs. 27c, 13a,b). The aesthetically favourable measured angle values often used to evaluate the shape and projection of the nose are recorded in the side view of my first diagrams of proportion (fig. 27c). In a harmonious nose, the angle between the nose and the forehead – the nasofrontal angle (NF) – is between 125 and 135 degrees, whereas the angle between the nose and the upper lip – the nasolabial angle (NL) – is set at between 90 and 120 degrees. The angle between the bridge of the nose and O – the meridian line (N–O) – should measure between 30 and 40 degrees (fig. 27c).

It is particularly interesting to note that when the basic diagram is applied to the Apollo of Piombino, it tallies perfectly with the canon of the above-mentioned proportions (fig. 28). The division of the face into three equally large horizontal sections is strictly observed in this sculpture. The width of the

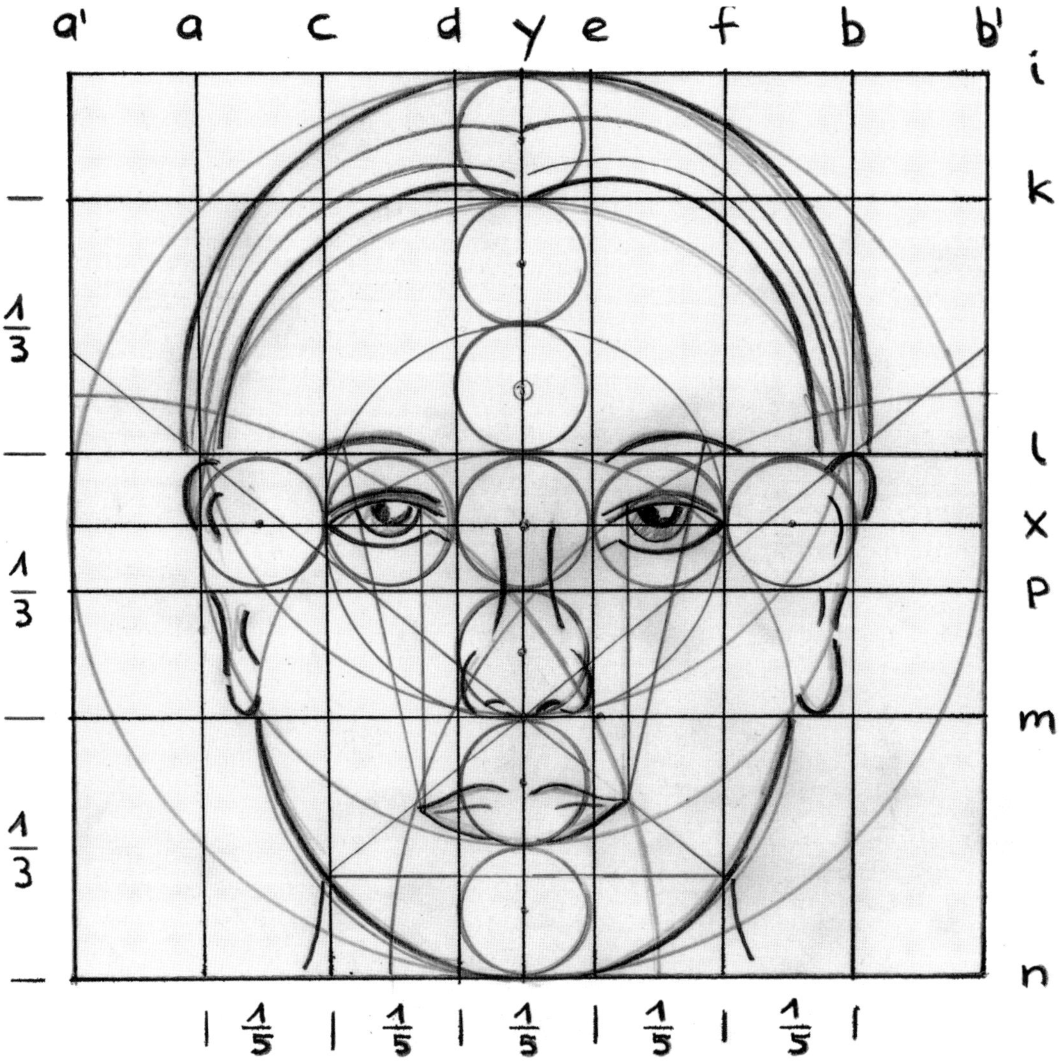

29

29 Studies of the proportions of the face, drawing by Urs Victor Burki

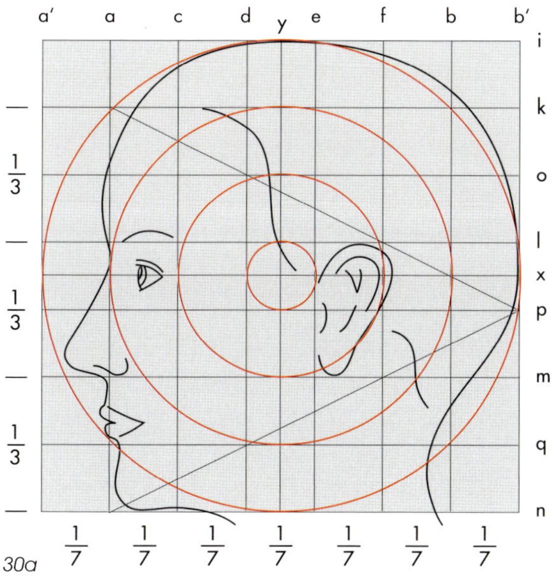

30a

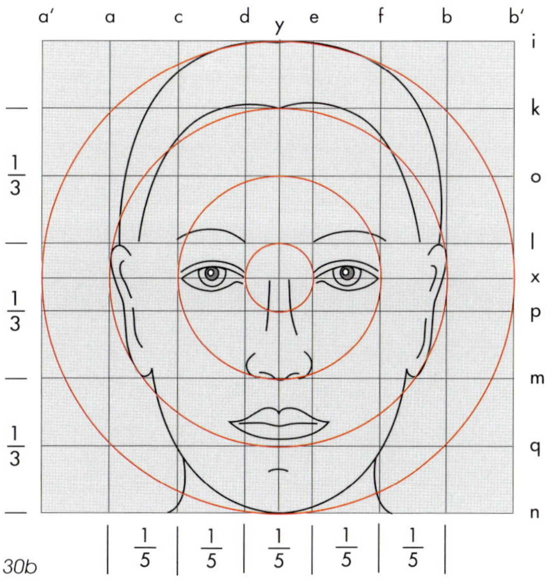

30b

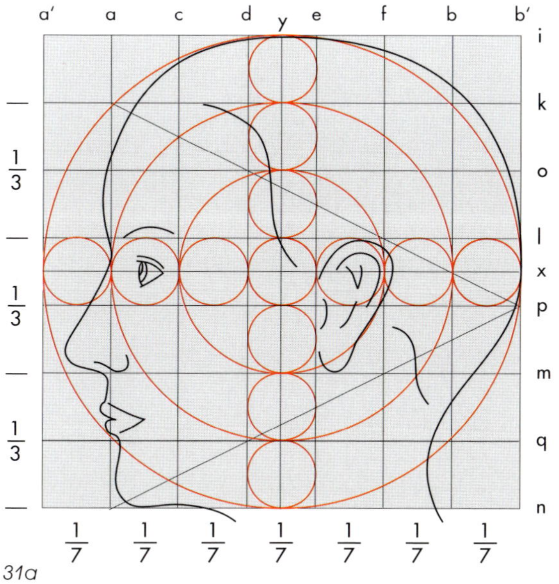

31a

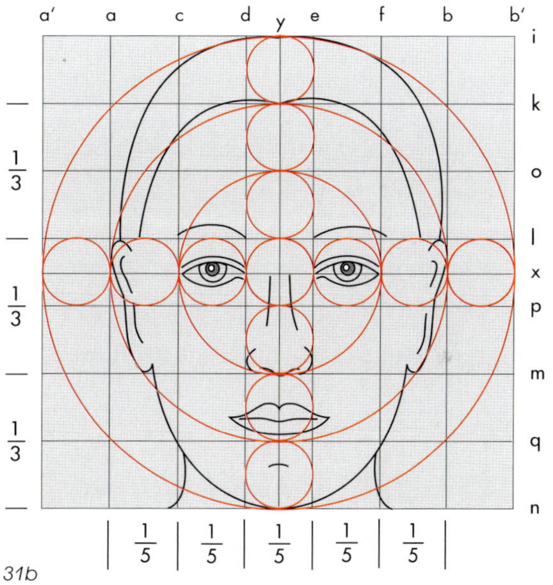

31b

30a Proportions of the face with central circles, profile, drawing by Urs Victor Burki

30b Proportions of the face with central circles, front view, drawing by Urs Victor Burki

31a Proportions of the face with central circles and vertically and horizontally drawn circles on axis x and y, profile, drawing by Urs Victor Burki

31b Proportions of the face with central circles and vertically and horizontally drawn circles on axis x and y, front view, drawing by Urs Victor Burki

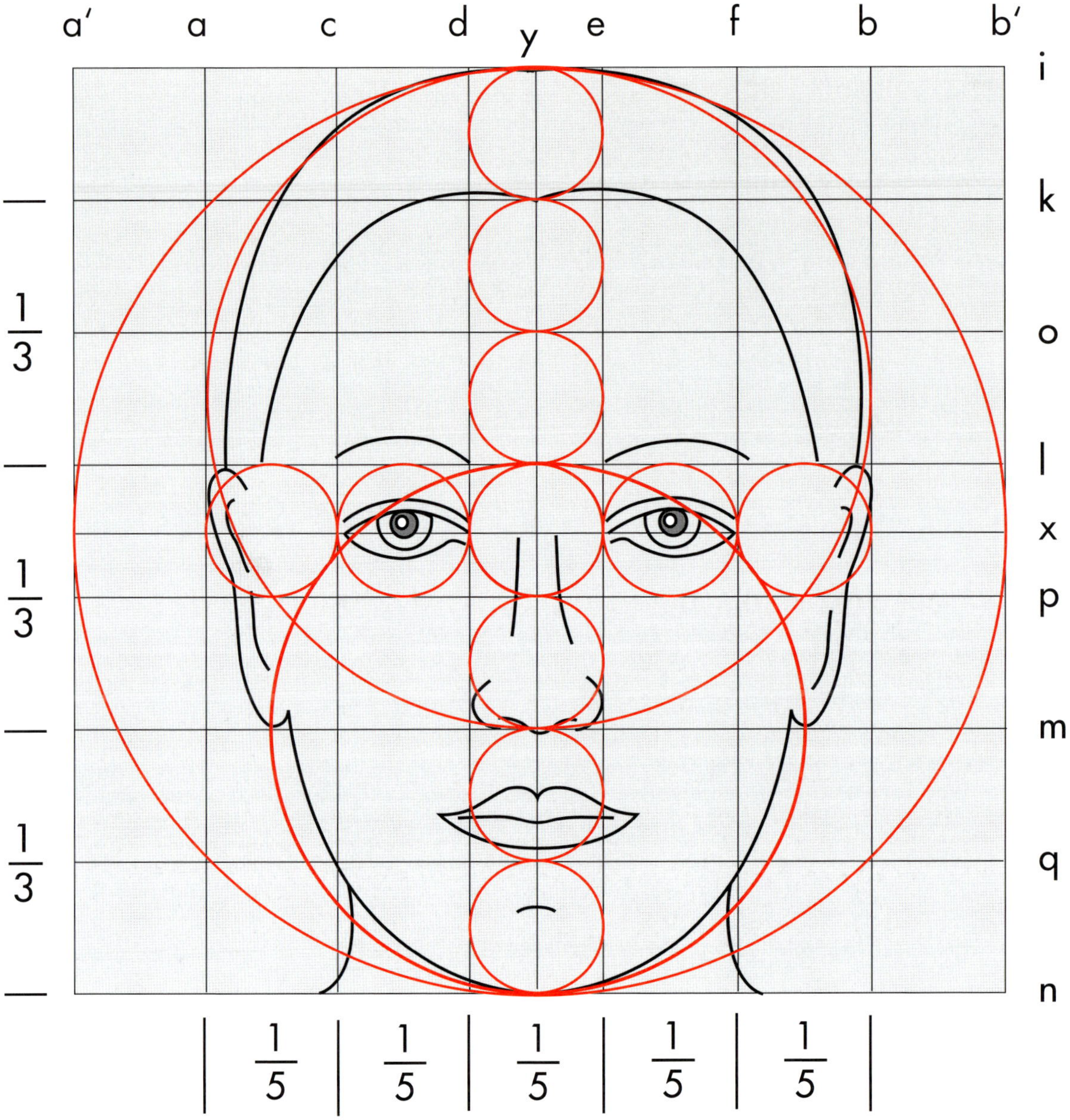

32

32 *Proportional diagram of the face by Urs Victor Burki*

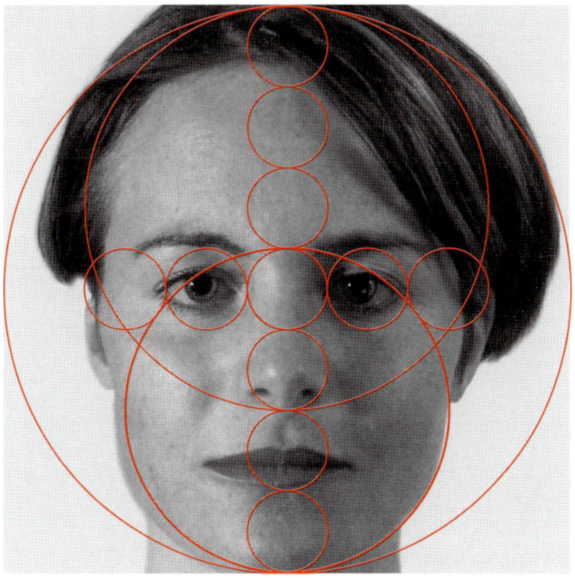

33a

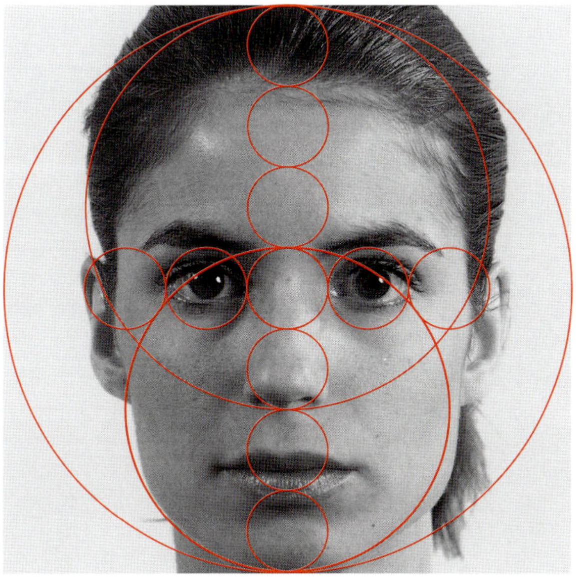

33b

eye corresponds to the distance between the eyes and the width of the nose. Interestingly enough, the face can also be divided into two at the level of the canthi (fig. 28).

The inclusion of additional lines and arcs of circles in my proportion studies pointed my investigations in a new direction (fig. 29). By way of additional illustration, I drew into my basic diagrams four arcs whose centres are located exactly at the centre of the square (figs. 30a,b). Since the sub-divisions of the face all consist of squares, I showed the horizontal and vertical subdivisions of the face additionally with seven vertically and horizontally drawn circles of equal size (figs. 31a,b). The centres of the vertically superimposed circles are located on the median line y. The centres of the horizontally adjacent circles are located on the median line x. In the front-view figure, the centrally-placed circle is as wide as each eye and is located in the upper half of the central third of the face (fig. 31b). The centre of this circle is also the centre of the outer circle, which touches all four sides of the square and thus the vertex and chin. The two circles located outside the middle circle have the same diameter as the width of the eyes, and the two outermost circles – which correspond to the outer one fifth of the face – end at the helix of the ear, on coordinates c, h.

At the centre of the third (counting from the top) of the seven equally-sized vertically drawn circles that subdivide the face horizontally is located the centre of a circle whose radius touches tangent i (vertex) and tangent m (base of the nose) and encompasses the upper half of the head over its whole width together with the region of the eyes and nose (fig. 32). In the middle of the base of the nose, at the point of contact of the second and third circles from the bottom, is located the centre of a circle which touches tangents n and l and encompasses the lower and middle thirds of the face. This coincides in the central third of the face with a part of the larger upper circle and encompasses the nose region and a part of the eye region (fig. 32).

Owing to the influence of the traditional sub-divisions of the face, which originate from painting and sculpture, the face is usually analysed by means of horizontal and vertical coordinates. The proportional diagram I have defined in the form of circles is particularly suitable for studying and

33a,b Photographs of faces with diagrams of proportions by Urs Victor Burki

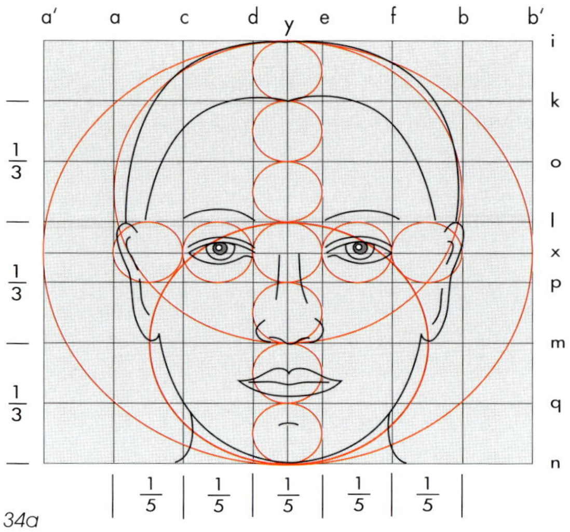

34a

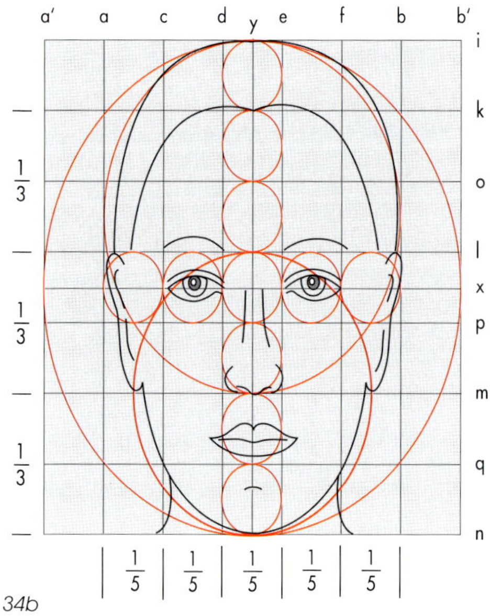

34b

analysing the proportions of the face and facial symmetry in the front view by accentuating the plastic shape of the face (figs. 33a,b). Relevant experience led me to take the view that it may be expedient for an aesthetic surgeon to incorporate these perspectives when considering how to render a face more beautiful and harmonious. Representing proportions with circles can, however, only be used for faces which can be subdivided with coordinates that are equally spaced from one another, both horizontally and vertically. If the face can only be subdivided with equilateral rectangles, it cannot then be divided up with contiguous circles of equal sizes. In the case of a longer head, it would be necessary to use ovals with a vertically oriented longitudinal axis, instead of circles; and horizontally oriented ovals in the case of a broader and shorter head (figs. 34a,b).

Even if these subdivisions of the face can serve as a pointer for judging the proportions and symmetry of a face, they can never be an absolute law for judging beauty. Even world-famous beauties with extremely harmonious-looking faces do not fit in every case the conventional, three-part division of the face into three equally-sized parts. For example, the upper third of Greta Garbo's face is slightly smaller than the lower two thirds and the central third of Marlene Dietrich's face is slightly larger than the upper and lower thirds. In the case of the Mona Lisa, the lower third of her face is significantly smaller than the central and upper segments, whereas in my adaptation of the Mona Lisa it is now only a few millimetres smaller than the central third of her face (figs. 35a,b).

In my comparative studies I also ascertained that the ear is rarely located exactly within the central third of the face, as in my studies of proportions and Leonardo's and Dürer's drawings of the proportions of faces. In most people the ear is larger than one third of the face and is lower than the nose; but quite often the ear is also higher than the nose and is seldom smaller than the latter. In

34a Proportions of the face with horizontally aligned ovals by Urs Victor Burki

34b Proportions of the face with vertically aligned ovals by Urs Victor Burki

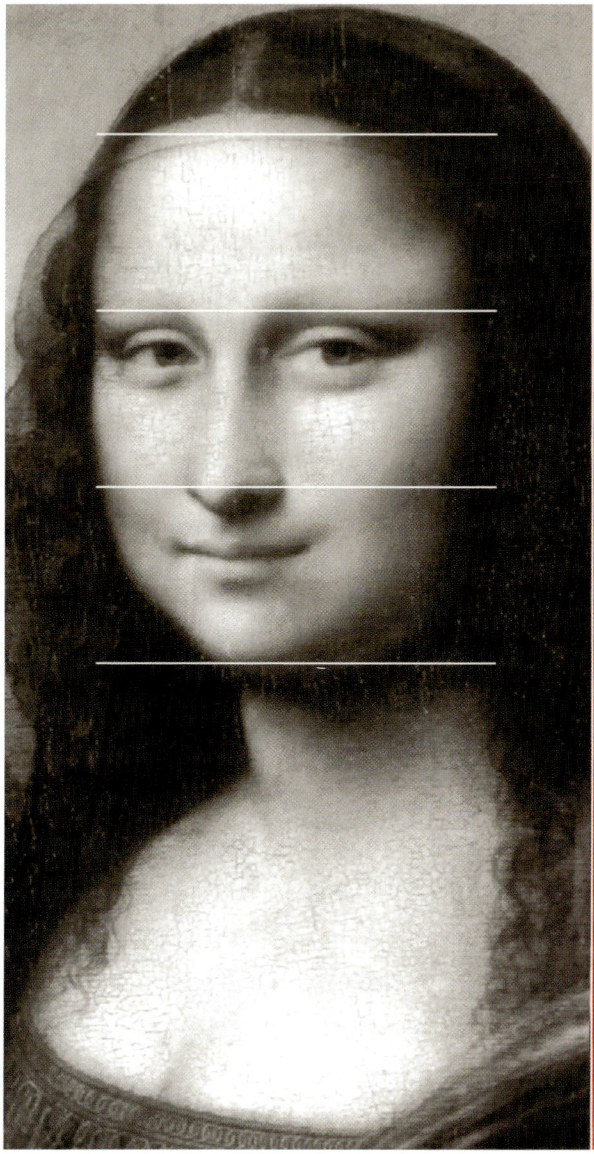

35a

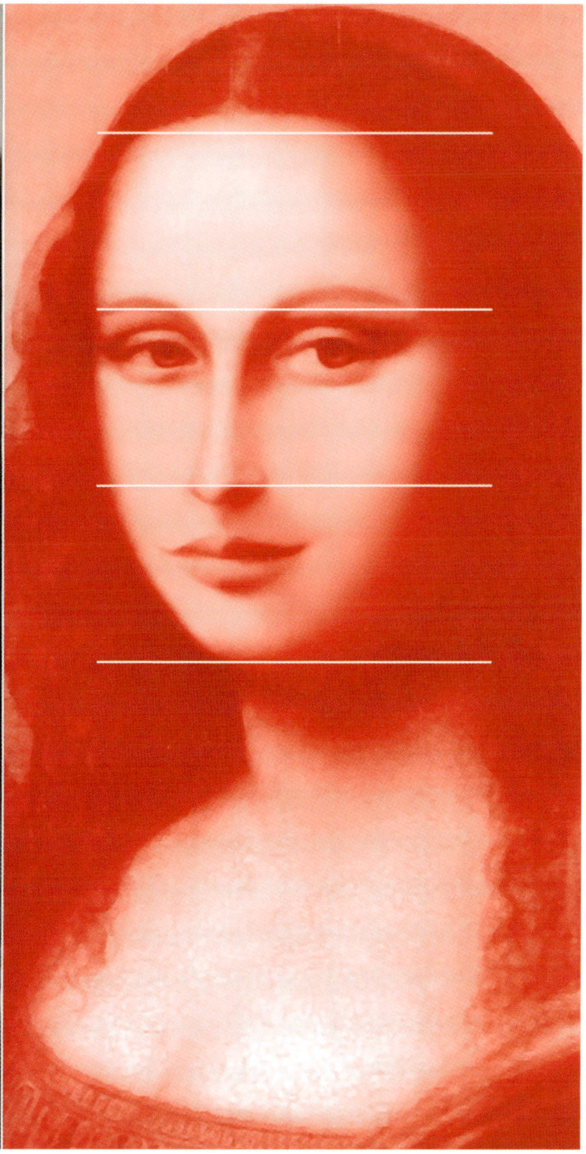

35b

35a,b Mona Lisa before and after aesthetic surgery with classical division of the face into three parts, study by Urs Victor Burki this context it is also worth mentioning that in many people the central third of the face becomes slightly smaller owing to the slight sinking of the forehead and eyebrow region, caused by ageing.

Golden Ratio and Fibonacci Sequences Applied to the Face

When searching for aesthetically favourable measured values and the laws of a harmonious face, I studied in depth the golden ratio (sectio aurea), which should contain a key to universal beauty. Although the Egyptians were already familiar with the golden ratio, it was described for the first time by the famous Greek mathematician and philosopher Euclid (330–270 BC) in his 6th book of the *Stoichea* (Elements) in around 300 BC. In this book Euclid noted that a line in the golden ratio is divided when the ratio of the whole line to the larger segment is the same as the ratio of the larger segment to the smaller one, or the ratio of the smaller segment to the larger one is the same as that of the larger segment to the whole line. The golden ratio can also be shown in a geometric construction (fig. 36). It results from the equations that the larger portion is 1.618... times larger than the smaller one and, conversely, that the smaller segment is 0.618 times smaller than the larger one. In mathematics this irrational number is the only one which yields its own reciprocal when the number one is divided by it: 1:1.618 = 0.618... It can also be obtained by its reciprocal plus 1 : 1.618... = 1 + 1/1.618... Moreover, it is the only number whose square to the right of the decimal point gives the same numbers: $1.618...^2 = 2.618...$ Mathematically, the golden ratio can be defined as follows: $1/2\,(1 + \sqrt{5})$.

The golden ratio is also referred to as phi or Φ after the Greek sculptor Phidias. Many Greek architects and sculptors applied the golden ratio. For example, many proportions of the Parthenon on the Acropolis correspond to the golden ratio. The human eye generally perceives proportions that obey the golden ratio to be harmonious and

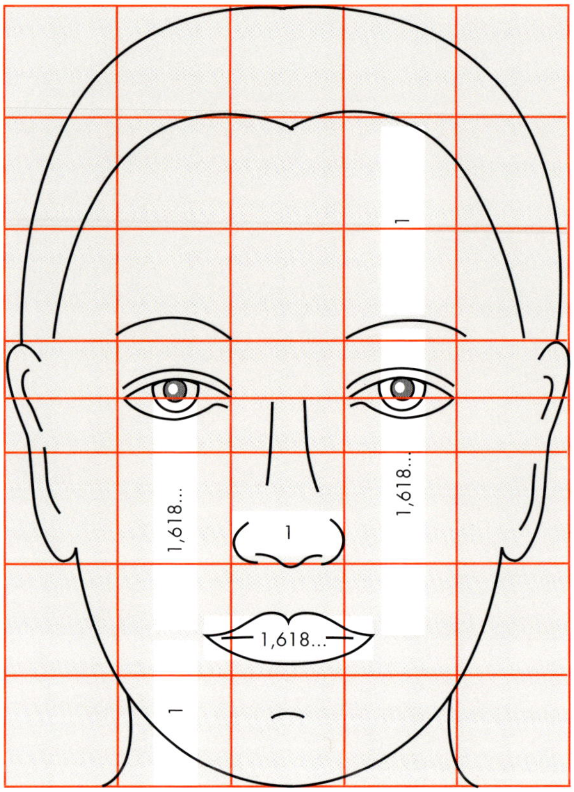

37a

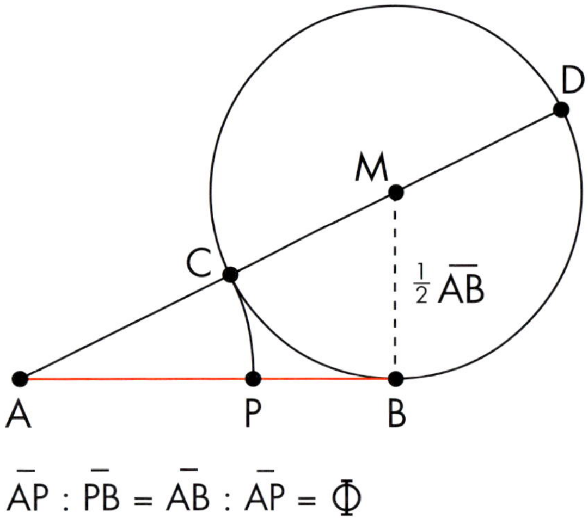

36

36 The golden ratio, geometric construction

37a Golden ratios applied to the face, drawing by Urs Victor Burki

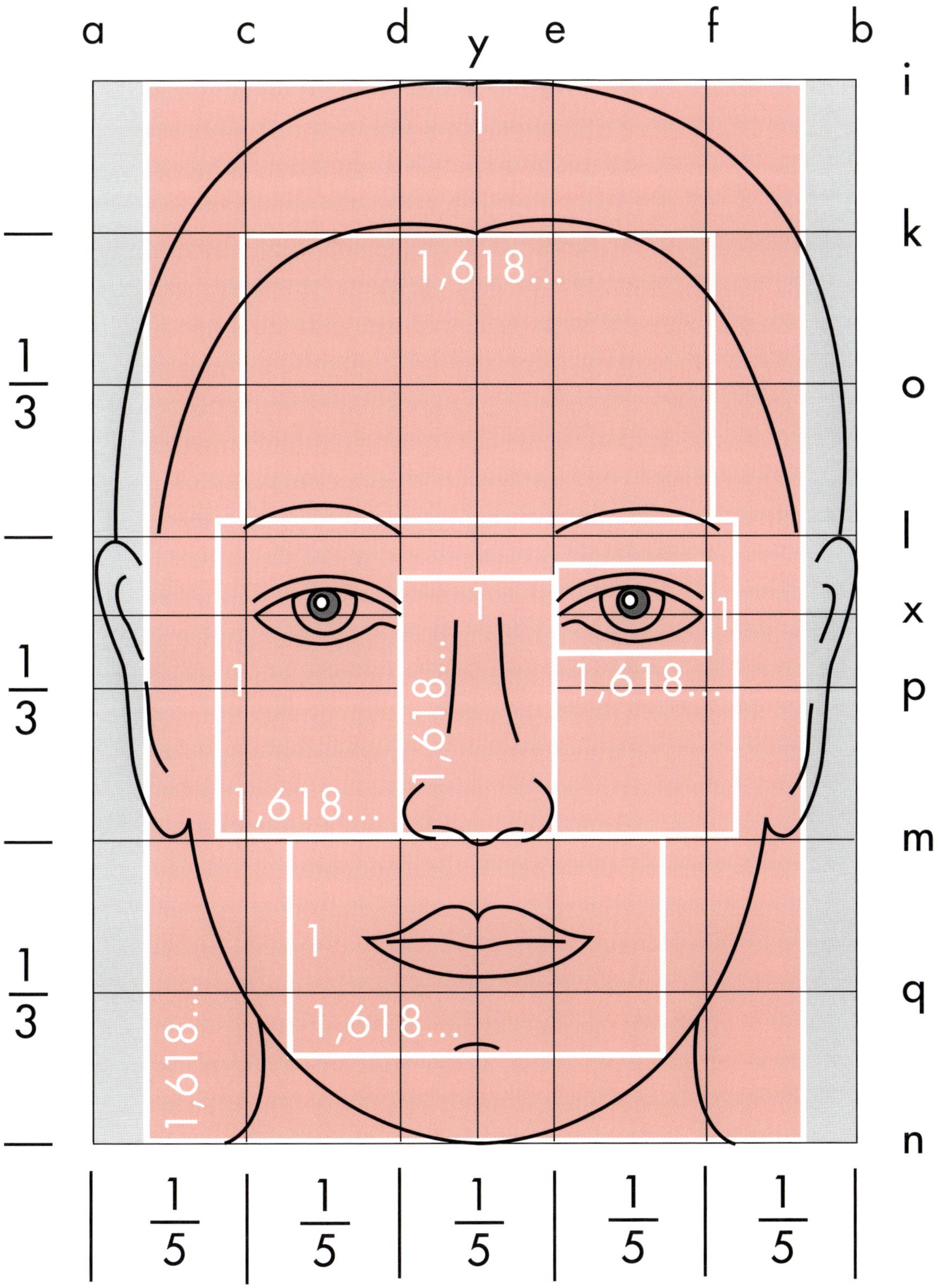

37b

37b Golden rectangles applied to the face, drawing by Urs Victor Burki

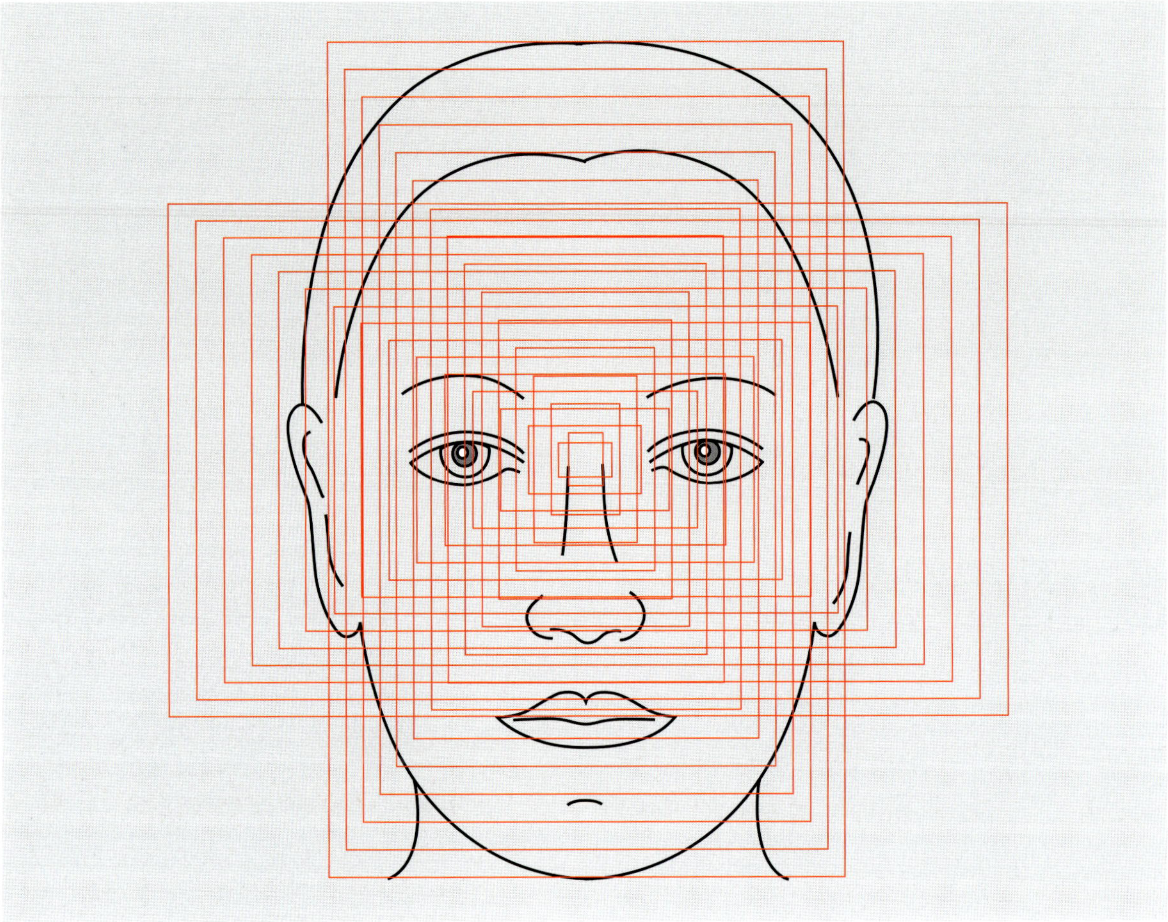

37c

37c Two series of golden rectangles applied to the face, study by Urs Victor Burki

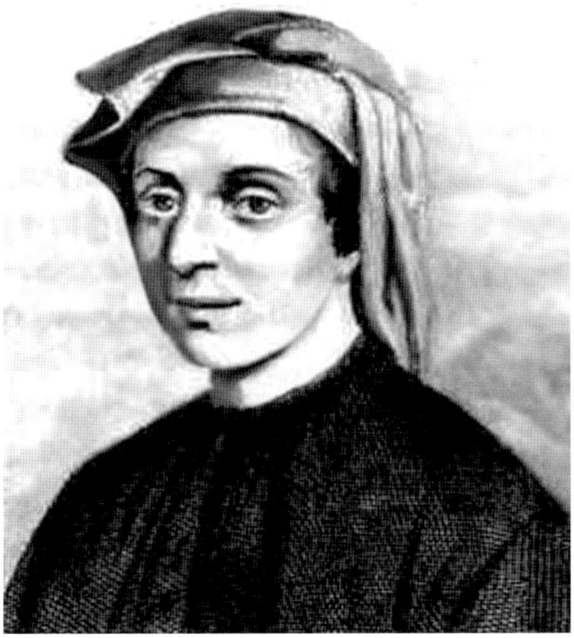

38

aesthetic. The eye is enabled to perceive unconsciously the golden proportions that are present everywhere in nature.

In the human body as well many parts are in a proportion to one another that corresponds to the golden ratio. The ratio of the upper to the lower part of the standing body, when divided at the height of the navel, corresponds to the golden ratio. The rules of the golden ratio also apply to the hand, where the ratio of the individual phalanxes to one another is as in the golden ratio: the proximal phalanx of each finger to the median phalanx and the median phalanx of each finger to its distal phalanx. The face also exhibits numerous "divine proportions". For example, the ratio between the width of the nose in the nostril region and that of the mouth and the ratio between the width of the eyes and that of the mouth corresponds to the golden ratio; or the distance from the frontal hairline to the eyebrow and the distance from the eyebrow to the middle of the mouth (stomion); or the distance from the middle of the eye (pupil) to the middle of the mouth (stomion) and the distance from the middle of the mouth to the lower edge of the chin (fig. 37a).

It is interesting to observe that the golden ratio in the face can be demonstrated not only in the form of golden proportions but also in the form of "golden rectangles", the ratio between the sides of which corresponds to the golden ratio. In many of the faces I analysed, the ratio of the height to the breadth of the head corresponds to the golden ratio. The same ratio between the sides is frequently also true of the nose, ear and also the eye, if the upper and lower eyelids are included in the measurement (fig. 37b). Using a series of juxtaposed "golden" rectangles of increasing size, which are projected onto individual regions of the face, many further golden ratios can be observed intuitively (fig. 37c). For example, I have drawn into my diagram "golden rectangles" in the region of the forehead, nose, eyes and mouth, as can be seen in the upper, middle and lower thirds of the face (fig. 37b). However, since these "golden rectangles" do not encompass any definite, clearly delimited areas of the face, they are not of great benefit for judging the harmony of a face. Facial analyses based on the golden ratio are therefore of less interest to aesthetic surgeons than to artists.

It is to the famous Italian mathematician Leonardo Fibonacci (1170–1250; fig. 38) also known as Leonardo Pisano or Leonardo de Pisa, that we owe the discovery of an interesting approximation to the golden ratio. Fibonacci's sequence starts with the number 1, which is first added to itself, then its product is systematically added to the preceding number of the sequence: 0, 1, 1, 2, 3, 5, 8, 13, 21, 34, 55, 89, 144, 233, 377, 610, 987 ... The new sum is always increased by a factor that tends to move closer to the golden ratio, 1.618... as the numbers grow larger. This sequence of numbers was defined by Fibonacci in the course of his mathematical research on the rate of reproduction of rabbits in subsequent generations. These numbers are often to be found in the plant and animal kingdoms; for example, the number of petals on a flower often

38 Leonardo Fibonacci, University of St. Andrews, Scotland

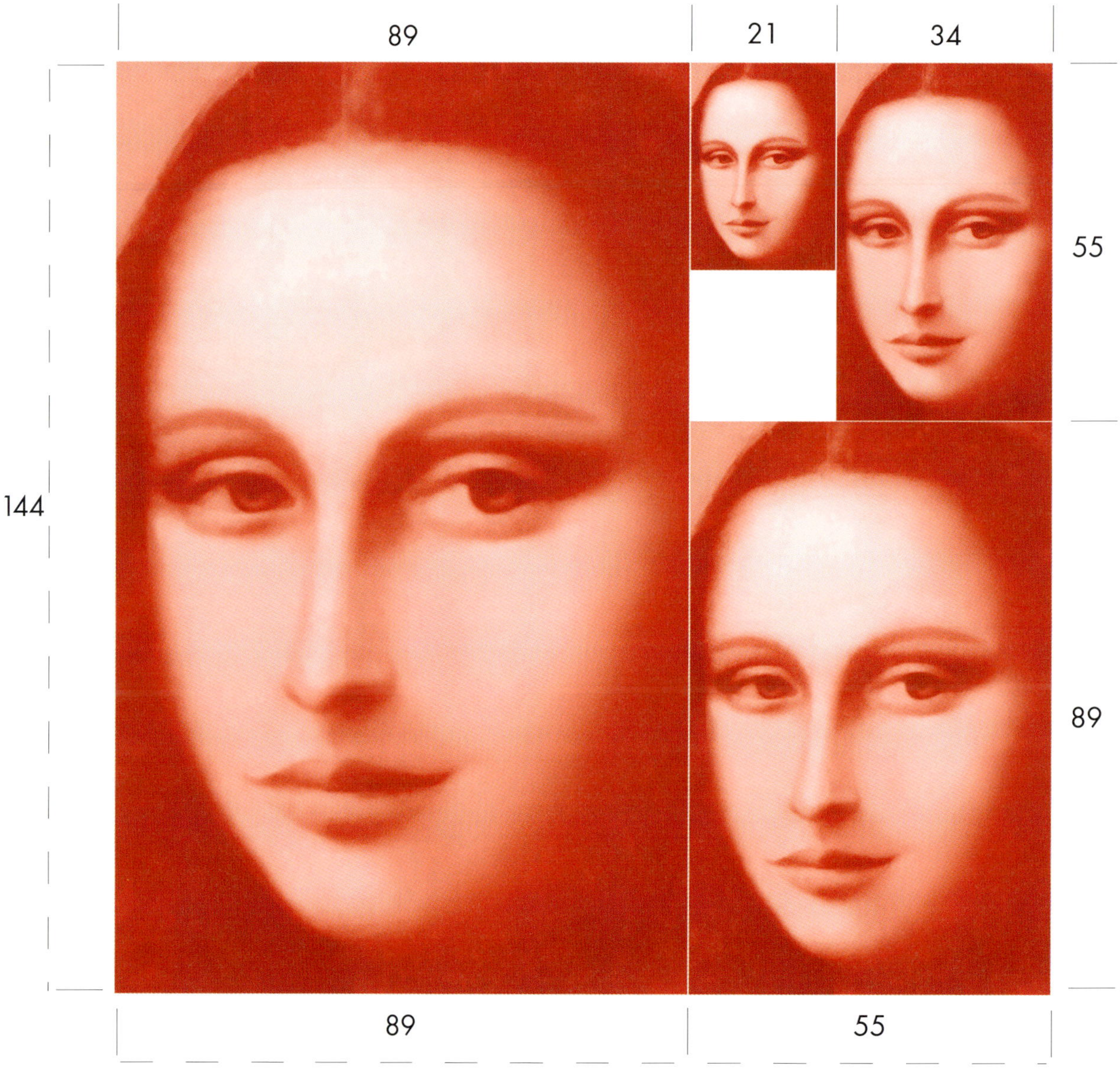

39a

corresponds to the Fibonacci sequence. This sequence also exists in the form of so-called golden spirals in snail shells and mussels and as spirals in plant seeds; sunflower seeds are also arranged in a spiral shape.

The figures showing "Mona Lisa after the aesthetic operation" illustrate very accurately the Fibonacci sequence and the golden spiral (figs. 39a,c).

My first figure shows the "Mona Lisa after the aesthetic operation" with golden rectangles, where the ratio of the larger to the adjacent smaller rectangle always corresponds to the golden ratio (fig. 39a). The golden spiral is constructed by drawing a quadrant into each square (fig. 39b). In the figure, which illustrates the golden spiral, the "Mona Lisa after the aesthetic operation" is reproduced in squares (fig. 39c). The ratio of the

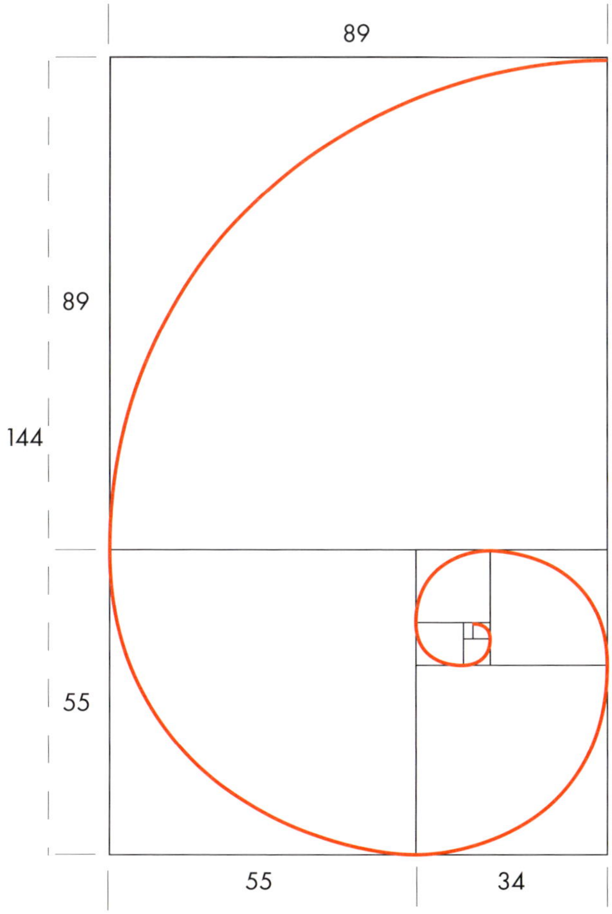

39b

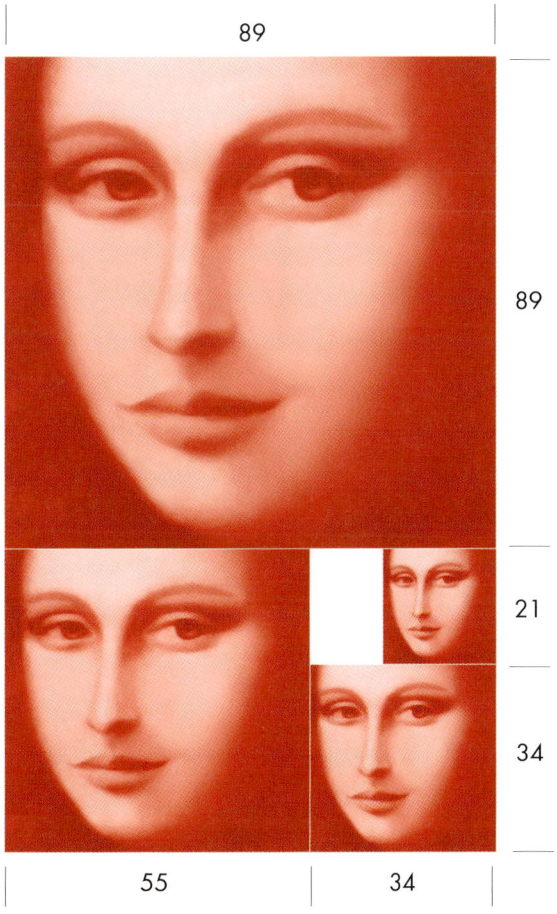

39c

larger to the next-smaller square corresponds to the golden ratio and the length of the sides of each square is equivalent to the sum of the sides of the two adjacent squares.

Symmetry of the Face: a Variable Factor

Ever since antiquity beauty has repeatedly been associated with symmetry. The wings of a butterfly, the six-point star of a snowflake, the stripes of a tiger or zebra – the beauties of nature appear to bear witness to an ever-present order, a symmetrical matrix of life. This order reigns even in the universe with its spherical heavenly bodies and the more or less symmetrical galaxies. The view according to which harmonious dimensions are created by a mirror-image counterpart has been widely held for centuries. The term "symmetry" was coined in 500 BC by the Greek sculptor Polycletus. What he called "sum metria" means nothing other than "even proportions".

Symmetry is extremely variable in the realm of aesthetics. When the part and counterpart are absolutely congruent, the overall picture may tip either way at any time and take on an expression

39a Sequence of the Fibonacci numbers with the Mona Lisa after aesthetic surgery, study by Urs Victor Burki

39b Golden spiral or Fibonacci spiral

39c Sequence of the Fibonacci numbers with the Mona Lisa after aesthetic surgery, study by Urs Victor Burki

of lifeless rigidity. An interesting experiment can be conducted with portraits of famous beautiful people and models. However, only faces that have been photographed absolutely frontally are suitable for this purpose. First of all, the face of the portrait is divided vertically into two equal-sized halves by a sagittal line. Then one should look at the position of the eyebrows, the shape and size of the eyes, the shape and size of the ears, the shape of the mouth and nostrils, etc. The differences between the left- and right-hand halves of the face are striking and significantly greater than would commonly be assumed.

No face is symmetrical and therefore the two sides of the facial profile are always different. This asymmetry is specific to each individual person and more or less pronounced, as the two profile photographs illustrate (figs. 40a,b). This phenomenon can be particularly well illustrated by synthetic images generated by a reflected, axial duplication – or "axial symmetry" – of the left or right half of the face (figs. 41a–d, 42a–d). This clearly shows how small asymmetries and irregularities lend expressiveness, originality and uniqueness to every face and make a significant contribution to its beauty.

Observer Distance Determines Facial Proportions

If one looks at one's face in a mirror from very close up, certain disharmonies – in particular those on which one's attention is focused – appear to be even more pronounced and by no means look the way someone viewing the face from a greater distance perceives them. The closer one moves to a mirror with one's face, the larger the nose appears, for example, compared with the rest of the face (fig. 43c). When one looks at one's face in a magnifying mirror, its proportions change even more and appear to be disharmonious (fig. 44).

It is a very interesting and rarely-observed fact that the proportions of the face alter according to

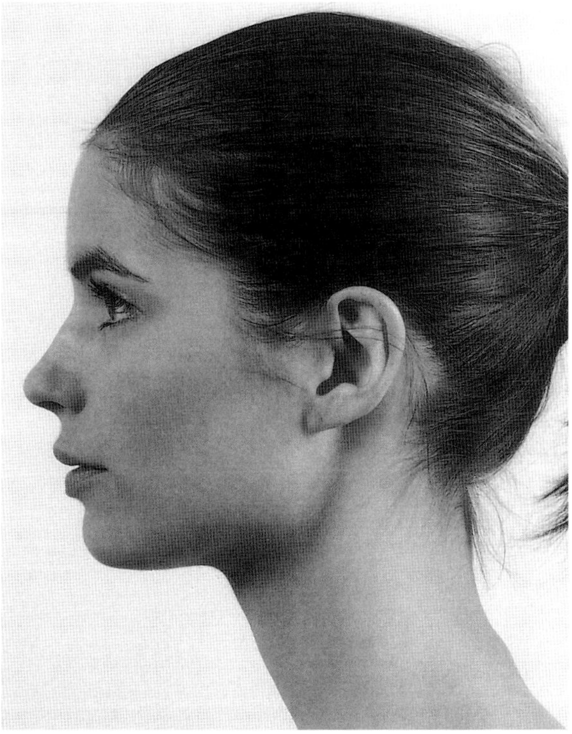

40a

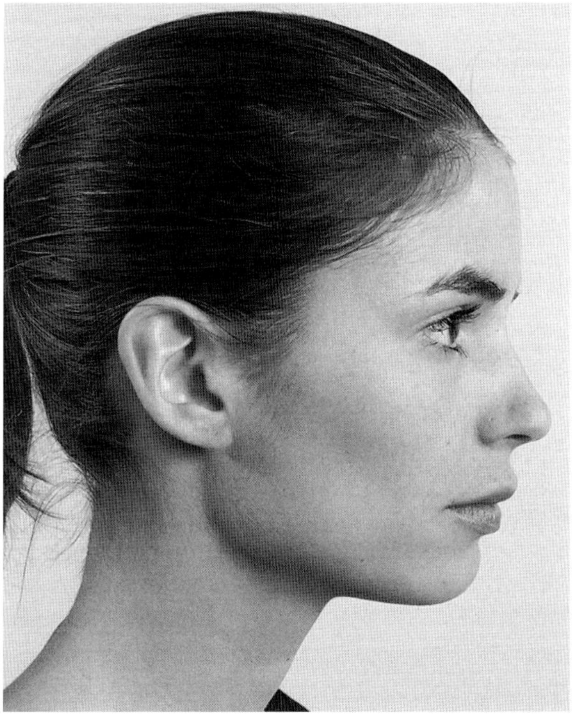

40b

40a Photograph of a woman's face, left profile
40b Photograph of a woman's face, right profile

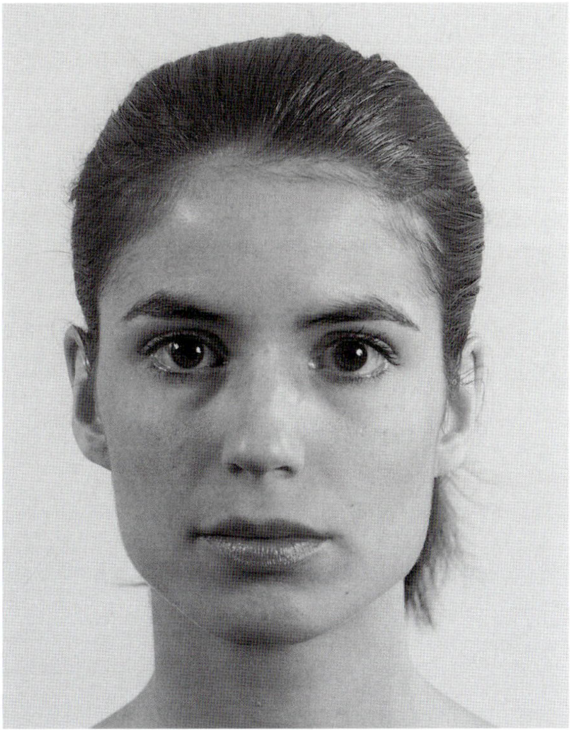

41a

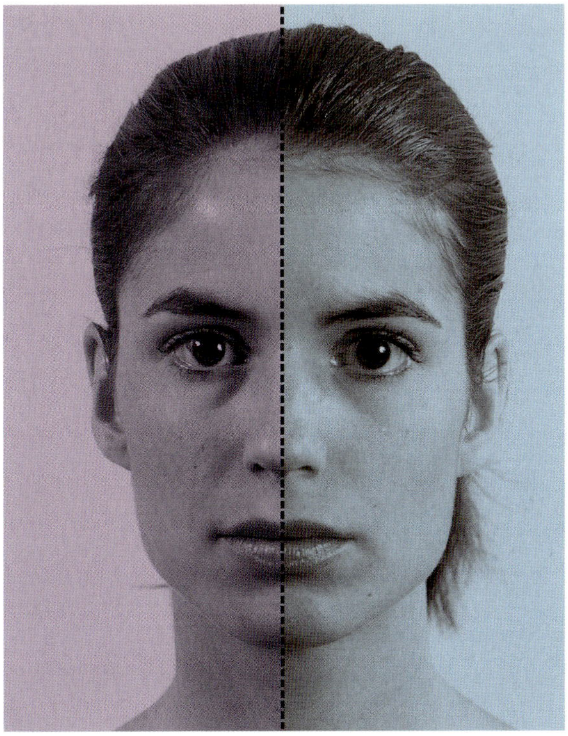

41b

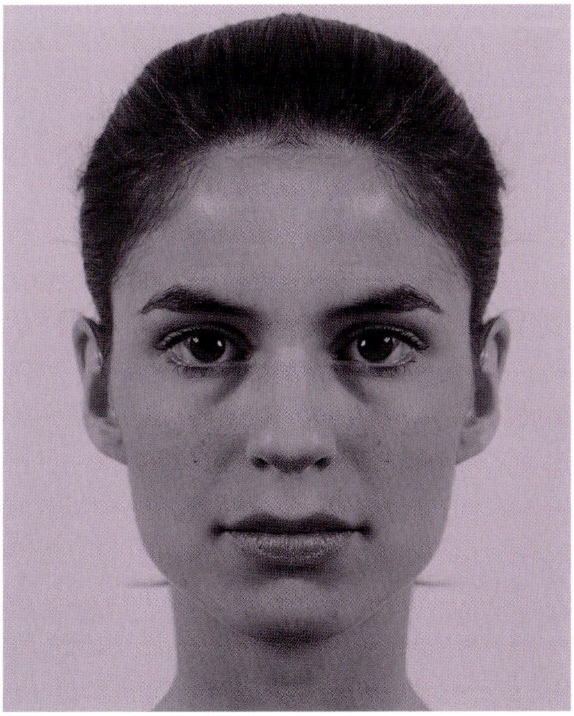

41c

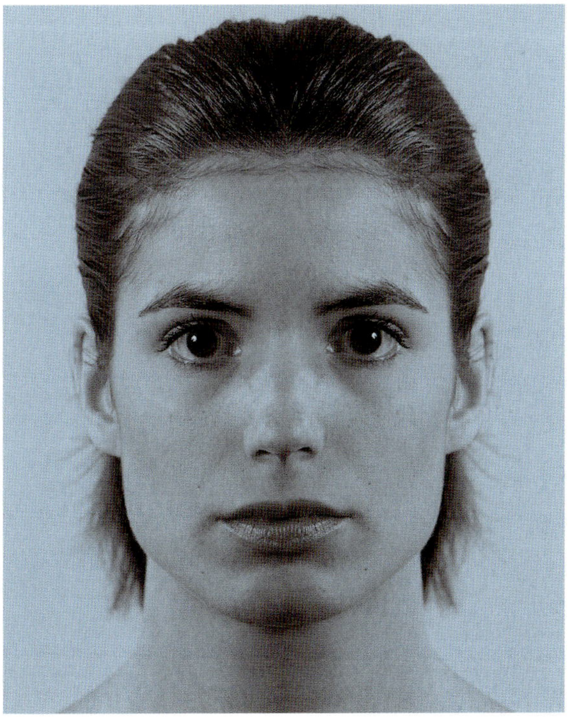

41d

41a Photograph of a woman's face, front view

41b Photograph of a woman's face, front view, with a central axis dividing the face into two halves, study by Urs Victor Burki

41c Reconstitution of the face by mirror duplication of the right half, study by Urs Victor Burki

41d Reconstitution of the face by mirror duplication of the left half, study by Urs Victor Burki

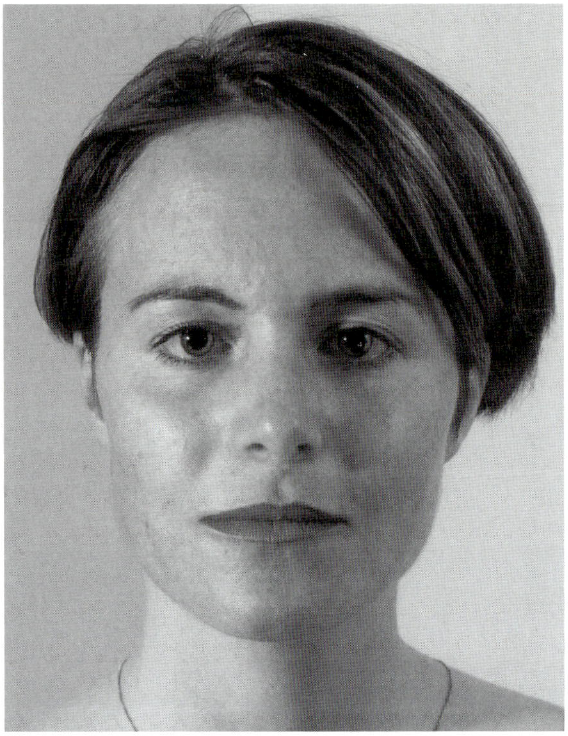

42a

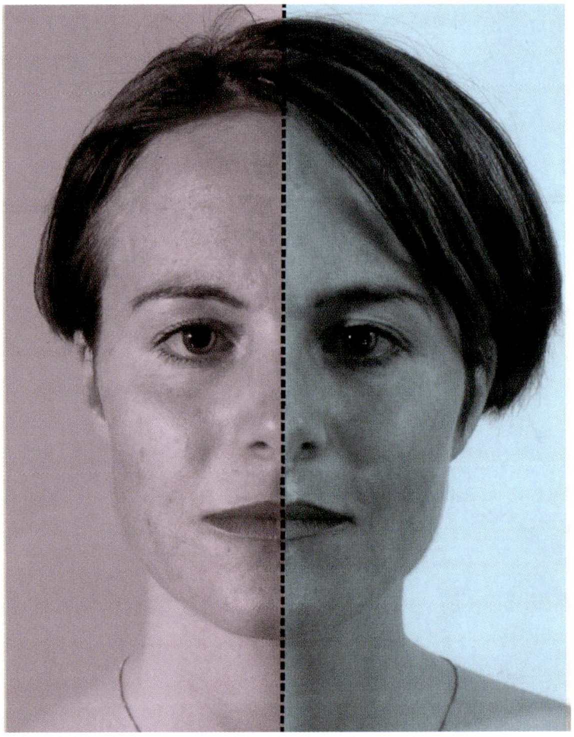

42b

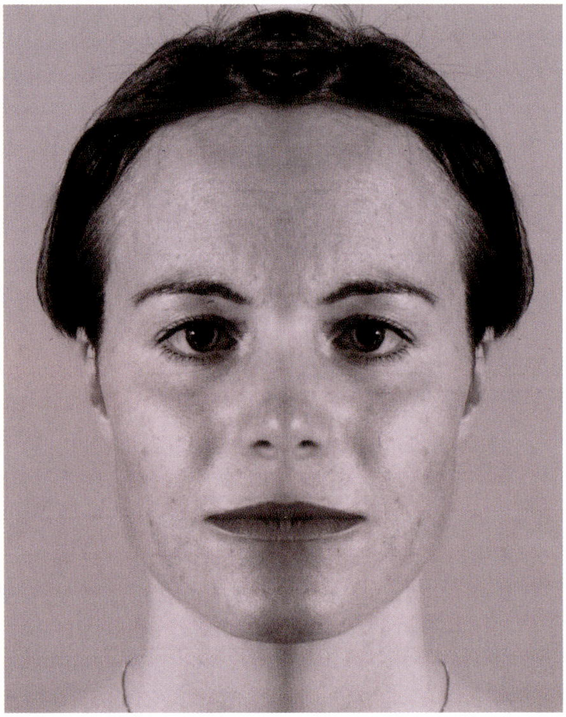

42c

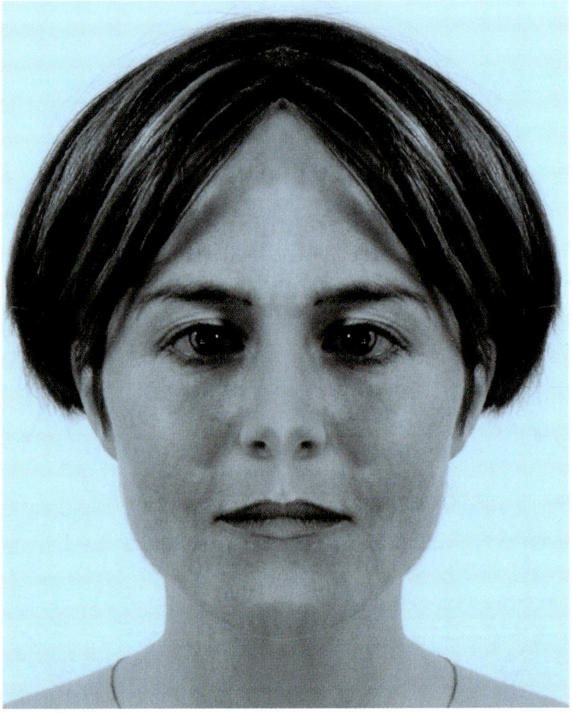

42d

42a Photograph of a woman's face, front view

42b Photograph of woman's face, front view, with a central axis dividing the face into two halves, study by Urs Victor Burki

42c Reconstitution of the face by mirror duplication of the right half, study by Urs Victor Burki

42d Reconstitution of the face by mirror duplication of the left half, study by Urs Victor Burki

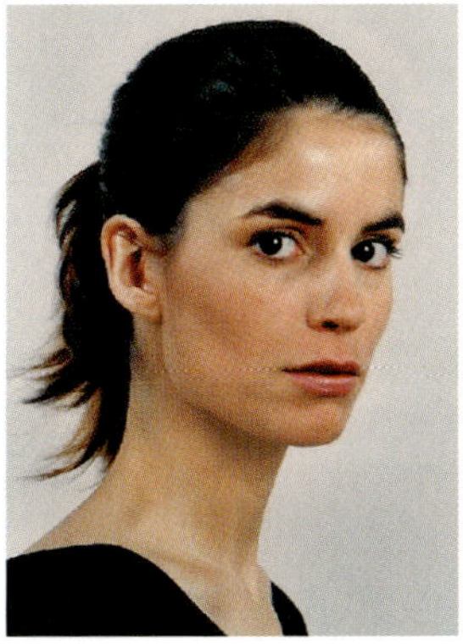
43a

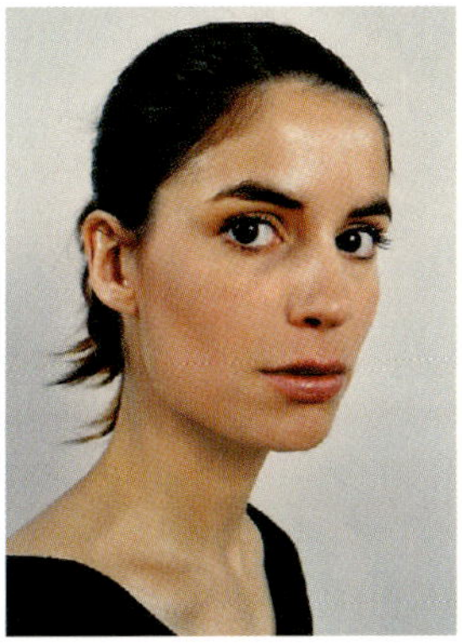
43b

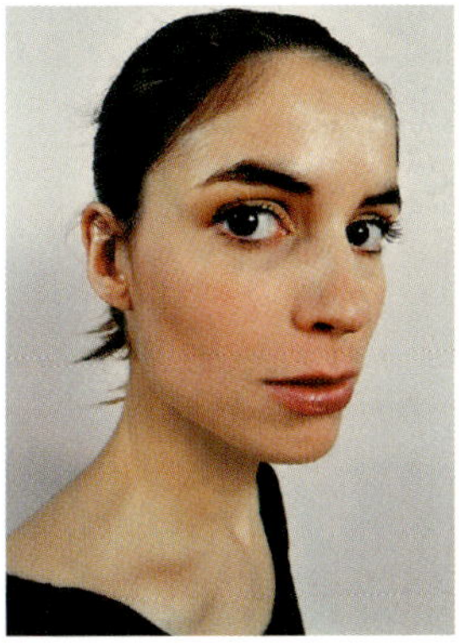
43c

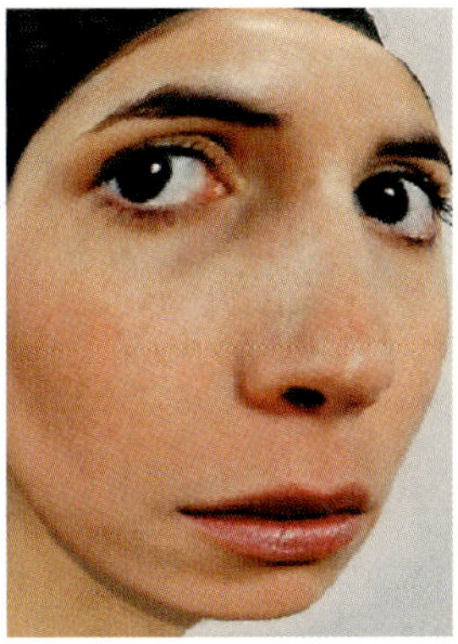
44

the distance from which it is observed, as is illustrated by the following photographs (figs. 43a–c). The young woman's face was photographed from the same angle, but with lenses of different focal lengths, which corresponds to different observation distances (figs. 43a–c). The face photographed with a lens of a focal distance of 50mm corresponds to an approximate observation distance of 100cm, the face photographed with a lens of 35mm to an observation distance of 60cm and the face photographed with a lens of 19mm to an observation distance of approximately 30cm (figs. 43a–c). The figures clearly illustrate that the proportions of the face viewed from very close up, from a distance of 30cm, differ so much from those of the face viewed from a distance of 100cm, that it is barely recognizable (figs. 43a,c).

Beauty Resides in the Eye of the Beholder

It is difficult to explain on which features the harmony of a face is really based. This human incapacity is explained by the fact that our eye takes in a far wider area than the ratio allows us to believe. One thing is certain: the beauty and harmony of a face are determined by the beauty of the individual facial elements and by a perfect interaction of all the individual parts with one another, together with personal radiance.

Although certain criteria required for a beautiful and harmonious face can be derived from proportional diagrams, they cannot determine either beauty or harmony in the human face. My personal conclusions concur with Albrecht Dürer's statement to the effect that no theory of proportions is capable of defining human beauty.

Leonardo da Vinci admirably summarized the phenomenon of facial beauty in his "Treatise on painting", addressed to the artists of his age. "Facial beauty can be equal in several persons, but the form will never be identical; and there are as many kinds of beauty as persons to whom it belongs."[4]

What is more subjective than beauty? Many authors maintain that beauty per se does not exist, but lies only in the eye of the beholder. Nevertheless fundamental aesthetic features, such as harmonious proportions, a balanced ratio between the individual parts of the face, and a certain degree of symmetry, have remained through the ages constant factors for a face perceived as beautiful and pleasing. That is why repeated attempts have been made to define beauty on the basis of a numerical system of ratios.

[4] *Leonardo da Vinci, "The problems of the painter", in: Sämtliche Gemälde und die Schriften zur Malerei, edited by André Chastel, Munich: Schirmer-Mosel 1990, p. 207*

43a Photograph taken with a 50mm lens for 24/36, equivalent to a distance of 100cm
43b Photograph taken with a 35mm lens for 24/36, equivalent to a distance of 60cm
43c Photograph taken with a 19mm lens for 24/36, equivalent to a distance of 30cm
44 Mirror with a magnification of about 2x

Pioneers of Aesthetic Facial Surgery

It is probably to the German practitioner Johann Friedrich Dieffenbach (1792–1847) that we owe the beginnings of aesthetic surgery.[1] He was regarded as the grand master of this discipline in the nineteenth century. His renown was so great that all the hospitals in Paris were made available to him when he came to operate in the French capital. He announced the various techniques he used in the case of partial reconstruction of the nose: to shrink the nostrils, he advised excising small, wedge-shaped pieces of skin and cartilage, and when the length or breadth of the nose had to be reduced, he used to remove fragments of skin on the outside, either vertically or horizontally.

The advent of modern rhinoplasty dates from 1887. At that time a New York surgeon, John Orlando Roe (1848–1919), published an article entitled the *The Deformity Termed 'Pug Nose' and its Correction by a Simple Operation*; it involved remodelling the tip of the nose from inside the nasal cavities.[2] In 1891 Roe described another operation, the purpose of which this time was to reduce the nose over its whole length.[3]

Another highly-talented surgeon, who was also to be a pioneer of rhinoplasty and later of facial aesthetic surgery, was the Berliner Jacques Joseph (1865–1934; fig. 1). On 11 May 1898 Joseph presented a case of rhinoplasty to the

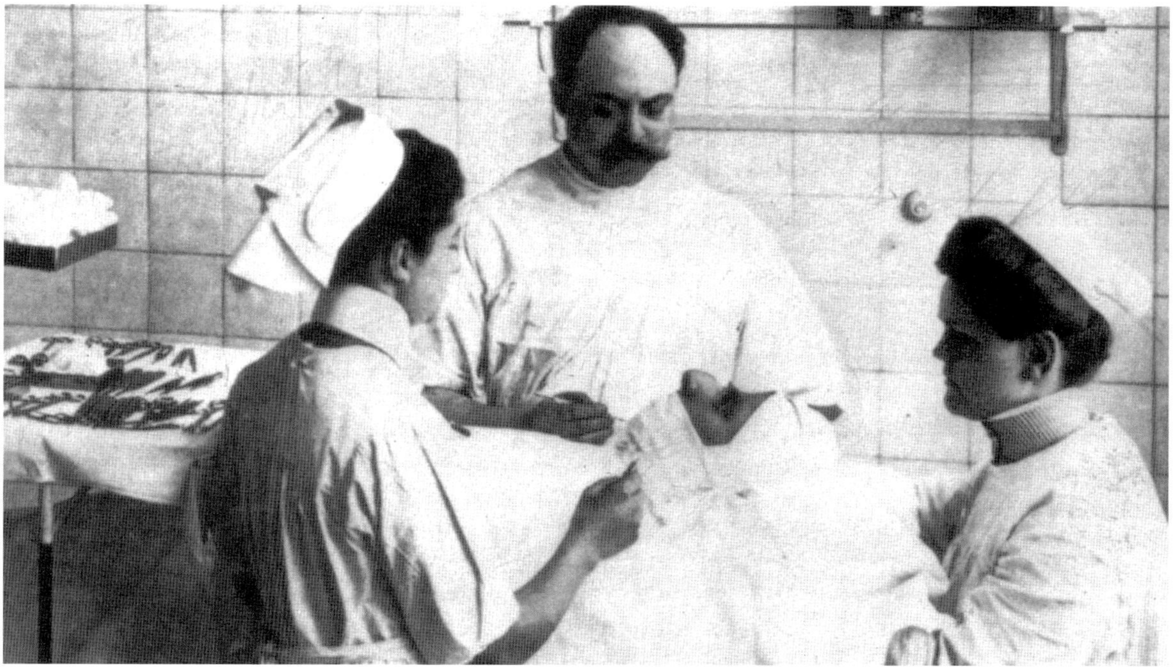

1

1 Jacques Joseph

Berlin Medical Society.[4] The patient was a 28 year-old landowner, afflicted by a prominent nose that caused him considerable embarrassment. Joseph showed photographs of the patient, taken before and after the operation (fig. 2). He had performed an external excision of the skin to remove the hump and shorten the nose. In 1902 he published a second article revealing that he had performed ten aesthetic operations of the same type.[5] It was not until about 1904 that Joseph declared he had used an internal method for his rhinoplasties.[6] At the time he had already completed 43 interventions. In 1905 he stressed the importance of photographs, which make it possible to study each patient's problems and to assess the postoperative results.[7]

The surgeon who is supposed to have performed the first facial rejuvenation operation came from Chicago: his name was Charles Conrad Miller (1880–1950; fig. 3). Some people called him a "visionary who was not afraid to go it alone"; others thought him an "impudent charlatan". In 1906 he wrote his first article on aesthetic surgery, more specifically on the excision of bag-like folds of skin from the eyelids.[8] One year later he brought out a book entitled *The Correction of Featural Imperfections*, the first book on aesthetic surgery.[9]

As Miller's book shows, the surgeon's career had already been well-established for several years. Charles Miller had opened his clinic on State Street in Chicago just after graduating from the Hospital College of Medicine in Louisville, Kentucky. He was then 23 years old. In the 1920 edition, Miller tells us about the improvement of his facial aesthetic surgery techniques.[10] He advised his colleagues to inform their patients in advance, to use a light-handed technique and sophisticated suturing material. The superiority complex he exhibited towards the medical profession, his patients and the public at large shows through the lines. He regarded his colleagues as narrow-minded and incapable of appreciating his remarkable intelligence.

The second practitioner who wrote about aesthetic surgery in medical history was called Fred-

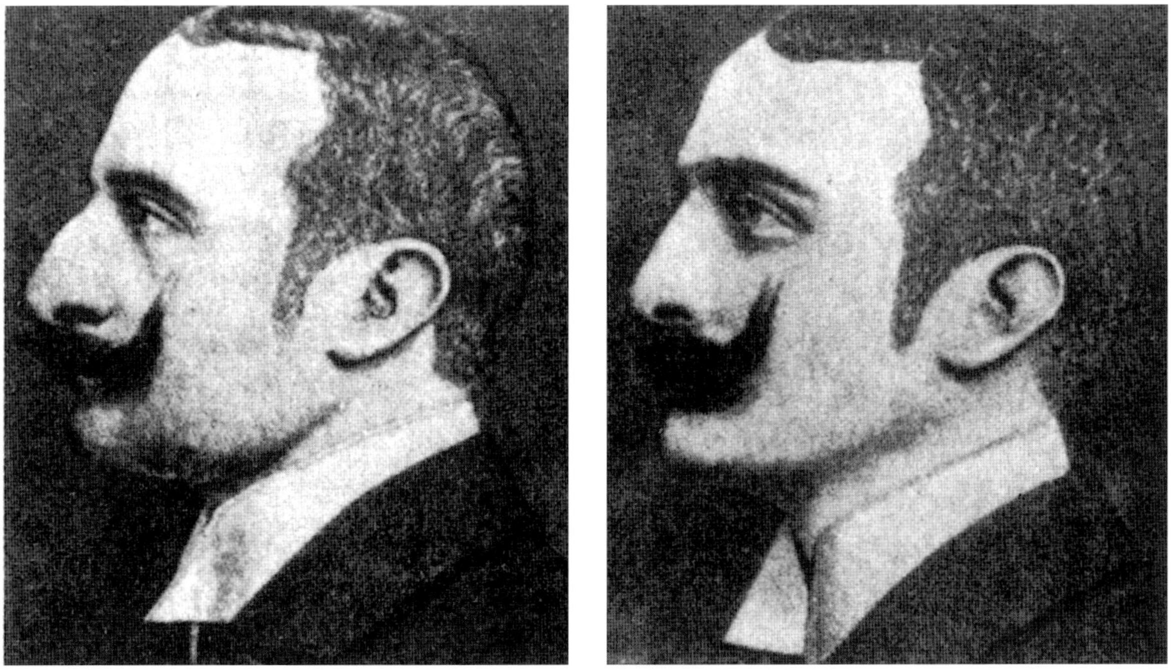

2

2 First rhinoplasty performed by Jacques Joseph with an external excision erick Kolle (1871–1929). This American of German origin practised aesthetic surgery in New York. In 1911 he published a book entitled *Plastic and Cosmetic Surgery*, a 500-page tome including 1522 illustrations.[11]

In 1912 a famous German surgeon, Eugen Holländer (1867–1932), wrote a treatise entitled *Aesthetic Surgery*, in which he explains how he had tightened the face of a Polish noblewoman and how the patient's female charm had played a key role in the operation.[12] Holländer had succumbed to "the art of female persuasion". To "refresh" the patient's face, he had removed a part of the skin on the hairline and in the natural folds. In the year of his death, in 1932, Holländer wrote that he had in fact performed this operation in 1901.[13] He had made an incision in the temporal region, going down to the pre-auricular fold around the ear.

In 1931 Erich Lexer (1867–1937), a Berlin surgeon, said he had never heard of face lifting when he performed this intervention on an actress in 1908. Before using his services, the actress had been in the habit of tightening the skin on her face at night by fixing strips of rubber above the dome of the skull. This technique, which the actress had applied for a long time, had caused transverse wrinkles that she wanted to have removed. Lexer maintained that a single operation would suffice. For this type of facelift, he made S-shaped incisions in the temporal region and behind the ears, as well as elliptical excisions on the forehead (fig. 4). He published a description of his interventions in a remarkable compendium entitled *Die gesamte Wiederherstellungschirurgie* (The whole of reconstructive surgery).[14]

A French surgeon, Raymond Passot (1886–1933), performed similar operations on the face. The article he published in Presse Médicale in 1919 was about the correction of facial wrinkles and was based on 14 cases.[15] Passot excised small segments of skin from different parts of the forehead, from the temporal region on the hairline, and in the vicinity of the ear lobe (fig. 8). He stressed the social value of these interventions and predicted that after an initial period of

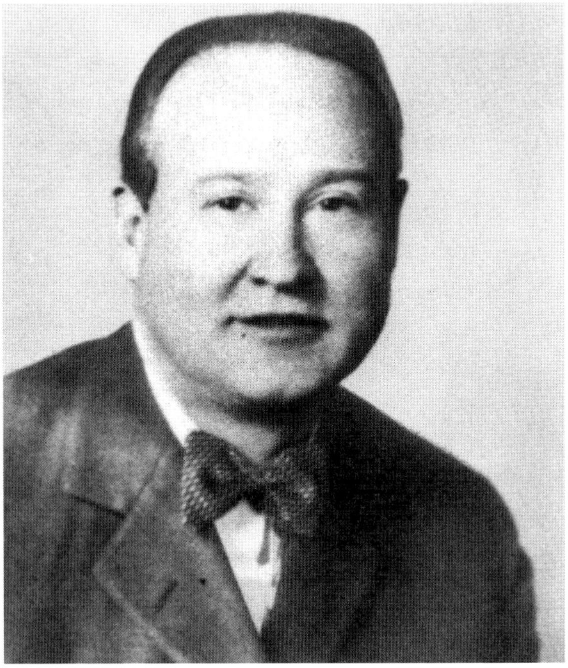

3

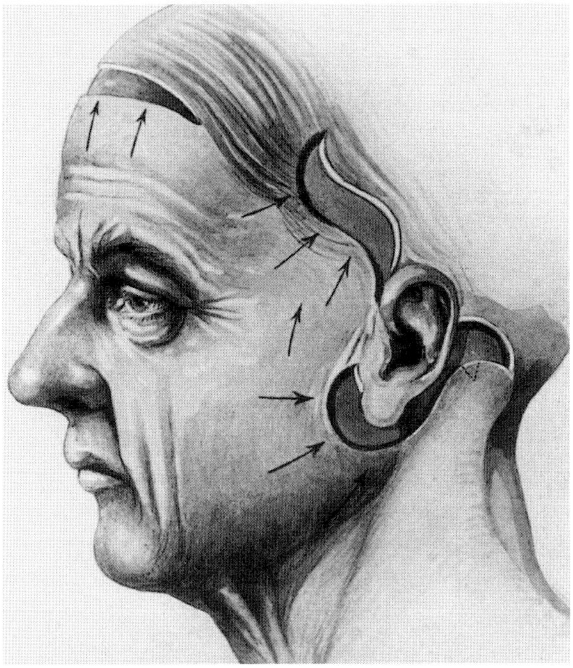

4

3 Charles Conrad Miller
4 Illustration of Lexer's operation

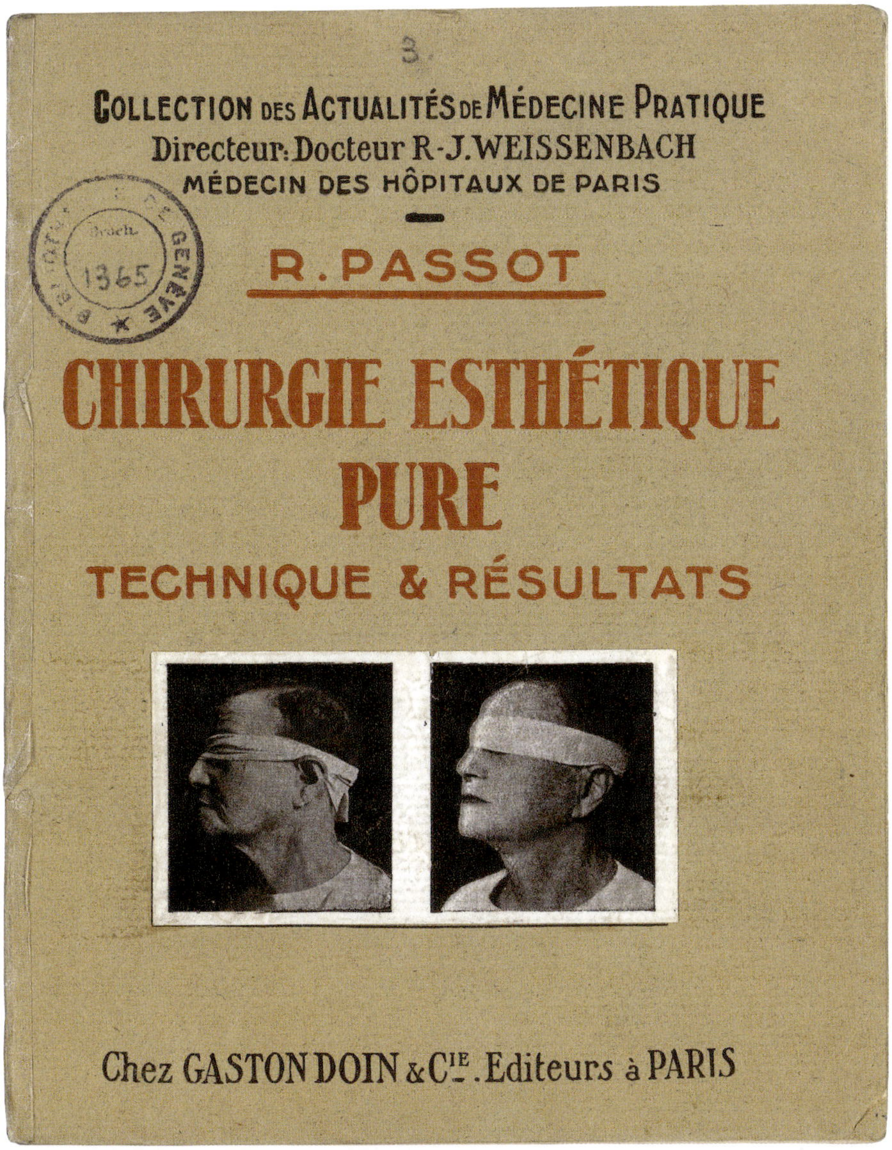

5

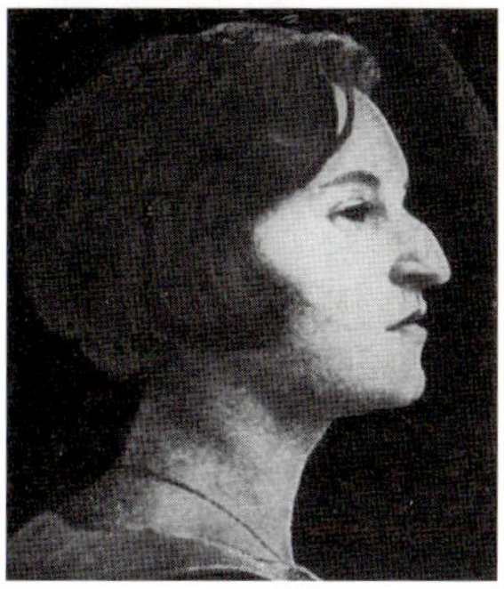

6a

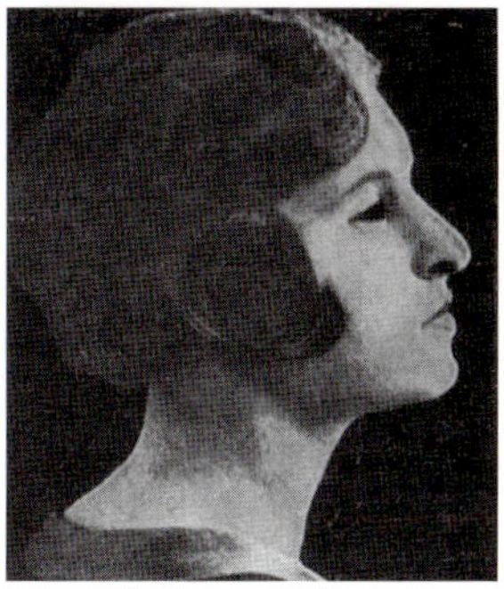

6b

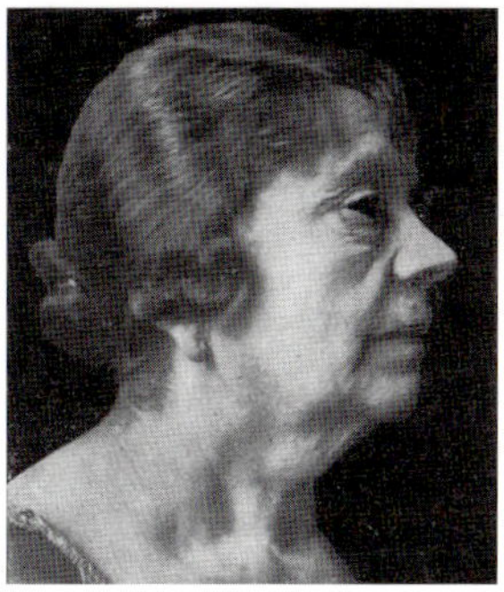

7a

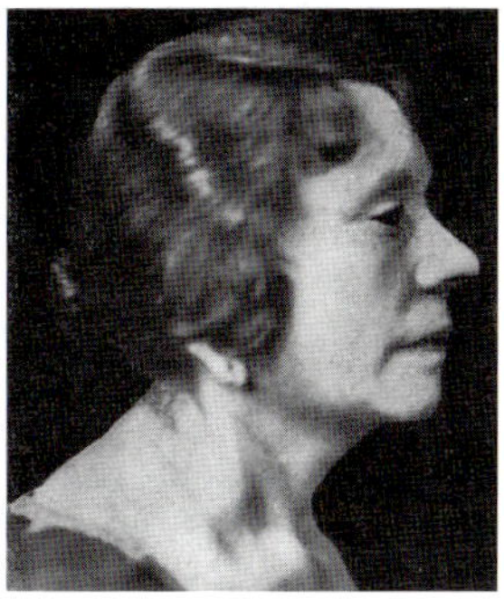

7b

5 Cover page of the book "Chirurgie esthétique pure", 1931, by Raymond Passot
6a,b Aesthetic rhinoplasty (before and after), performed and commented by Raymond Passot, 1931[18]
7a,b Face and neck lift (before and after), performed and commented by Raymond Passot, 1931[19]

scepticism, aesthetic surgery would become unanimously accepted by the public and the medical profession.[16] The Academy of Medicine reacted very negatively and advised him to stop this type of activity, which it considered to be frivolous. But Passot took no notice of their warning. After having practised nothing but aesthetic surgery for 11 years, in 1931 he published a description of more than 3,000 facial rejuvenation operations in a book entitled *Chirurgie esthétique pure* (Pure Aesthetic Surgery) (figs. 5, 6a,b, 7a,b).[17,18,19]

He emphasized in particular the value and importance of aesthetic surgery compared with plastic and reconstructive surgery: "It is here that the exclusive specialization of the aesthetic surgeon who has known hundreds or thousands of similar cases is likely to make the patient feel confident."[20] In the same book Passot mentions the cardinal role of the preliminary examination. He thinks it is as important as the operation itself: "This is where the aesthetic surgeon must show artistic taste and psychological insight."[21] Further on, he describes at length the various disfigurements encountered, stressing the importance of aesthetics and natural harmony: "The surgeon's task is not to destroy the facial expression: Lavater rightly defended this theory a century ago: the facial features are not spare parts that have been put together by chance. (...) So there we have the first commandment of pure aesthetic surgery: do not modify an organ radically; correct the excessiveness of the tendencies; deem them unaesthetic only when they begin to destroy harmony; always allow the traces to remain and do not alter the meaning of a physiognomy by a standard transformation or alteration."[22]

Passot was also the first to emphasize the importance of the choice of anaesthesia for his patients: "All these interventions can be performed using local anaesthetics, a fundamental point which must be stressed, as this method will allow the patient to return to work straight away; in such cases one should not expose the patient to risk: although the risk of an accident caused

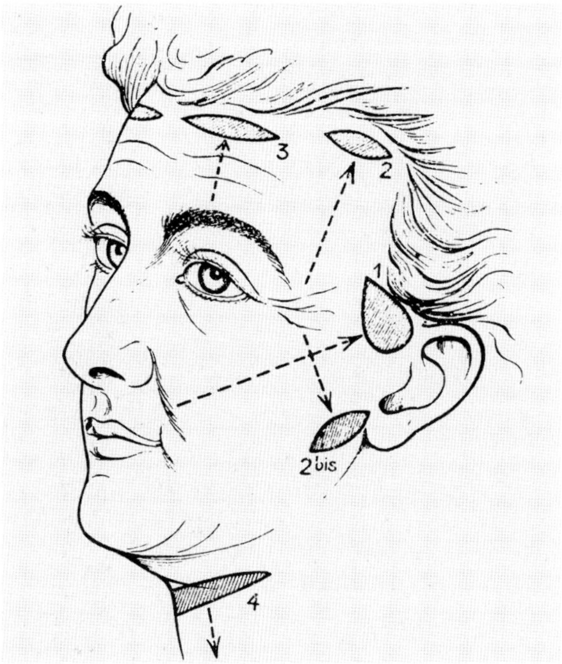

8

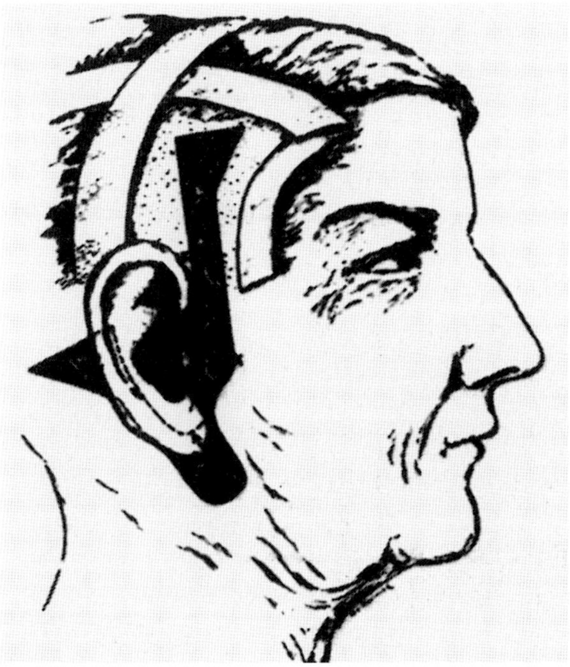

9

8 Segmentary excision of skin according to Passot's technique
9 Joseph's face lifting technique in 1928

by anaesthesia is very low, it demands that we formally require local anaesthesia."[23]

Adalbert Bettmann (1883-1964) of Portland, Oregon, was probably the first to take photographs of his patients before and after a facelift. He published them in the medical literature in 1920[24], and also showed for the first time a very wide incision, extending from the temporal region to just in front of the ear, beneath and behind the lobe. These incisions were very similar to those made today for a conventional facelift.

Shortly afterwards, in 1921, Jacques Joseph published some photographs of his patients' faces before and after their facelift.[25] Joseph's skin incisions are very similar to those described by Bettmann, but the results appearing on the photographs seem far superior. Proceeding in stages, he operated first one side of the face, then treated the other a few weeks later. According to his own accounts, in 1912 he performed a facelift on a 48-year-old woman who was complaining of premature ageing, which she blamed for the failure of her business activities.

Although most of Joseph's patients belonged to the aristocracy and the acting world, he was the first plastic surgeon to emphasize the psychosociological aspects of aesthetic surgery. He focused mainly on the first wrinkles appearing on the face, which are liable to be an obstacle to career women aged between forty and fifty. It was an entirely new concept in the literature of aesthetic surgery. At the time, the University of Leipzig considered this discipline immoral and Joseph, who was passionately devoted to it, was temporarily suspended from his academic positions. But far from being discouraged, he continued to develop new surgical techniques (fig. 9). He was soon to enjoy an international reputation and trained numerous surgeons around the world. In 1928 he published a book entitled *Nez et autres plasties du visage* (Nose and other plastic surgery of the face), which was truly a landmark treatise on facial aesthetic surgery.[26]

This overview of the origins of facial aesthetic surgery would not be complete without mentioning one of the most remarkable figures in the field, Suzanne Noël (1878–1954; fig. 10). She was the first woman to devote herself exclusively to aesthetic surgery. She operated in Paris in her apartment, which she had converted into a private clinic. Her operations were all performed using local anaesthesia. Her patients were mainly famous people, actresses or aristocrats. Before deciding which corrective method she was going to use, Dr. Noël used to give her patients an idea of the final result by drawing their skin taut with specially adapted tweezers. She

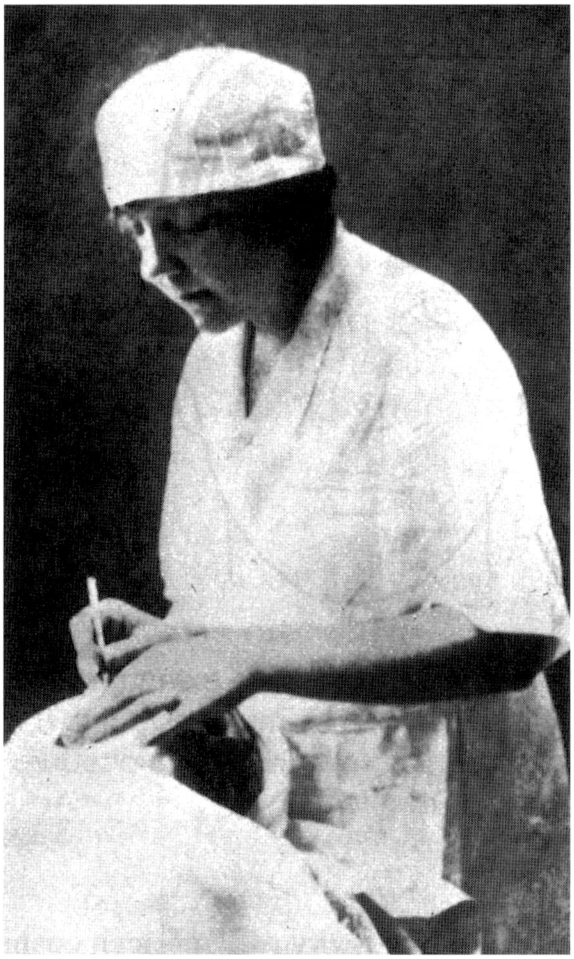

10

10 Suzanne Noël, the world's first woman to perform aesthetic surgery

adjusted the direction and extent of skin tightening to suit her patients' wishes. Elliptical incisions on the hairline were one of her specialities; she also did pioneering work in face lift and eyelid surgery. In a book published in 1926 and entitled *La Chirurgie Esthétique: Son Rôle Social* (Aesthetic surgery: its social role), she emphasized the psychological impact of aesthetic surgery.[27] The book contains descriptions of the new surgical techniques employed, as well as 59 pre- and postoperative photographs, showing the quality of the results obtained. It was common knowledge that Suzanne Noël had herself undergone multiple face lift and eyelid operations.

I would like to close this brief outline with a photograph from Suzanne Noël's book about the social role of aesthetic surgery. It shows a patient who just had a face lift under local anaesthesia in the practitioner's small clinic. She has put on her hat and is drinking a cup of tea before going home. Her affable smile and the trust she radiates symbolize the beneficial effect produced by this fascinating branch of surgery on the patients' well-being (fig. 11).

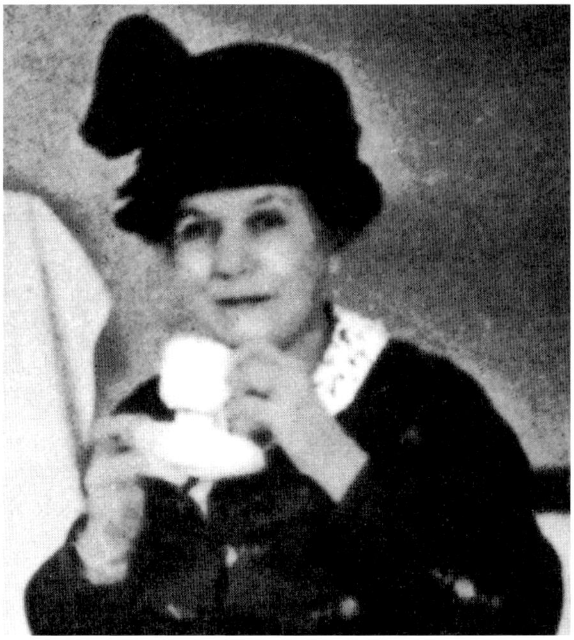

11

The aim of this chapter was to review briefly the first experiments in the field of aesthetic surgery. The principal defect of these long-established face lifting techniques was that they did not provide for skin detachment. Subsequently, numerous improvements were made in this area (skin detachment, tightening of the deeper tissues, etc.), and a wide range of complementary techniques was developed (endoscopic surgery, laser resurfacing, liposuction, chemical peel, filling, etc.), so that today a well-understood rejuvenation technique produces better, much more harmonious and longer-lasting results, with invisible scars.

It was only later that the medical profession recognized the importance of rejuvenation surgery for the patients' psychological and physical well-being. But even though aesthetic surgery today still encounters sometimes certain prejudices, it is generally no longer considered frivolous. It is now accepted that a person may choose to improve their appearance and, with it, their quality of life.

11 Patient operated under local anaesthesia by Suzanne Noël, drinking a cup of tea after her face lift operation

[1] Johann Friedrich Dieffenbach, *Die Operative Chirurgie*, F. A. Brockhaus, 1845

[2] John Orlando Roe, *The Deformity Termed 'Pug Nose' and its Correction by a Simple Operation*, in: Medical Record, vol. 31, 1887, p. 621, re-published in: Plastic Reconstructive Surgery, vol. 45, 1970, p. 78

[3] John Orlando Roe, *The Correction of Angular Deformities of the Nose by a Subcutaneous Operation*, in: Medical Record, vol. 40, 1891, p. 57

[4] Jacques Joseph, *Über einige weitere Nasenverkleinerungen*, Berliner Klinische Wochenschrift, 1902, p. 851

[5] Jacques Joseph, *Nasenverkleinerungen"*, Deutsche Medizinische Wochenschrift, vol. 30, 1904, p. 1095

[6] Jacques Joseph, *Intranasale Nasenhöckerabtragung*, Berliner Klinische Wochenschrift, 1904, p. 650

[7] Jacques Joseph, *Weiteres über Nasenverkleinerungen*, Münchner Medizinische Wochenschrift, vol. 52, 1905, p. 1489

[8] Charles C. Miller, *The Excision of Bag-like Folds of Skin from the Region about the Eyes*, Medizinischer Brief, vol. 34, 1906 p. 648

[9] Charles Conrad Miller, *The Correction of Featural Imperfections*, Oak Printing Co., Chicago, 1907

[10] Charles Conrad Miller, *Cosmetic Surgery, The Correction of Featural Imperfections*, F. A. Davis, Philadelphia, 1925

[11] Frederick Kolle, *Plastic and Cosmetic Surgery*, D. Appleton and Co., New York, 1911

[12] Eugen Holländer, *Die Kosmetische Chirurgie*, in: Joseph, M. (ed.): Handbuch der Kosmetik, Verlag von Veit, Leipzig, 1912, p. 688

[13] Eugen Holländer, *Plastische (Kosmetische) Operation: Kritische Darstellung ihres gegenwärtigen Standes*, in: G. and F. Klemperer, (ed.): Neue Deutsche Klinik, vol. 9, Urban und Schwarzenberg, Berlin, 1932, pp. 1-17

[14] Erich Lexer, *Die gesamte Wiederherstellungschirurgie*, vol. 2., J. A. Barth, Leipzig, 1931, p. 548

[15] Raymond Passot, *La chirurgie esthétique des rides du visage*, in: Presse Médicale, vol. 27, 1919, p. 258

[16] Raymond Passot, *La correction chirurgicale des rides du visage*, Bulletin de l'Académie de Médecine, vol. 82, 1919, p. 112

[17] Raymond Passot, *Chirurgie esthétique pure (technique et résultats)"*, G. Doin & Cie, Paris, 1931

[18] Operation before and after, performed and commented by Raymond Passot: a) "Young woman presenting a hyperconvex nose (osteocartilaginous kyphosis)". b) "The corrective operation consisted of endonasal ablation of the prominent osteocartilaginous tissue (local anaesthetic)". In: Raymond Passot, *Chirurgie esthétique pure*, G. Doin & Cie, Paris, 1931, p. 8

[19] Operation before and after, performed and commented by Raymond Passot: a) "Aging woman; pronounced sagging in the face and in the neck." b) "Temporal and periauricular incision; detachment of the facial and cervical integuments; two deep sutures, one attaching the buccinator muscle, the other attaching the exterior margin of the platysma; suture concealed in the hair and retroauricular skin fold. Radical corrective procedure. " In: Raymond Passot, *Chirurgie esthétique pure (technique et résultats)*, G. Doin & Cie, Paris, 1931, p. 3

[20-23] Raymond Passot, *Chirurgie esthétique pure (technique et résultats)*, G. Doin & Cie, Paris, 1931, pp. 3 – 10

[24] Adalbert Bettmann, *Plastic and Cosmetic Surgery of the Face*, Northwest Medical Journal, vol. 19, 1920, p. 205

[25] Jacques Joseph, *Hängewangenplastik (Melomioplastik)*, Deutsche Medizinische Wochenschrift, vol. 47, 1921, p. 287

[26] Jacques Joseph, *Nasenplastik und sonstige Gesichtsplastik*, Leipzig: Curt Kabitzsch, 1931

[27] Suzanne Noël, *La chirurgie esthétique: son rôle social*, Masson et Cie, Paris, 1926

The illustrations in this chapter are from the article "The Development of Aesthetic Plastic Surgery: A History", Blair O. Rogers, M.D., in: The Creation of Aesthetic Plastic Surgery, reproduced with the author's permission.

Aesthetic Facial Surgery

Facial Rejuvenation Surgery

It is the face that carries the most apparent traces of ageing. By adulthood, we have established an ideal image of our self, an image we always have in mind even as we age, because it conveys our identity (fig. 1d). Rejuvenation procedures bring us at least part way back to this self-image, creating the illusion that years have literally been restored (figs. 1a–d). It is not uncommon that the achieved external rejuvenation imparts greater self-confidence and a new feeling of well-being, while acting as a genuine source of harmony.

In recent decades various aesthetic surgery techniques have been developed to counteract the effects of ageing, and in the last few years some extraordinary progress has been made in the field. Today aesthetic facial surgery offers much more safety and accuracy. When it is practised by expert hands, complications are extremely rare and never of a serious nature. Aesthetic rejuvenation surgery is in general much more individualized and the results are more natural-looking and longer-lasting than in the past. The emphasis is on re-countering as well as tightening. Countering means shifting or moving underlying tissues in different areas of the face and the neck. Various new methods have also been developed to smooth the skin surface.

Sometimes only a relatively minor intervention such as a lipo-injection (micro lipofilling) or eyelid surgery (blepharoplasty) is indicated for the rejuvenation of the face. Often it may be necessary to combine different procedures (facelift, blepharoplasty, micro liposculpture, dermabrasion, chemical peeling etc.), always with the objective to garantee the best possible result. The ultimate aim is to always achieve a significant rejuvenation consistent with naturalness.

Deciding on the right time for facial rejuvenation is a very individual matter. Facial rejuvenation surgery can be considered when the skin and the underlying tissues start to sag or deposits of fat and deeper wrinkles appear.

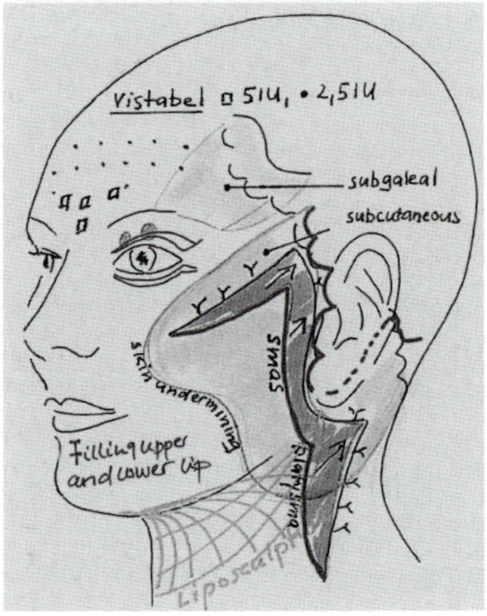

1a

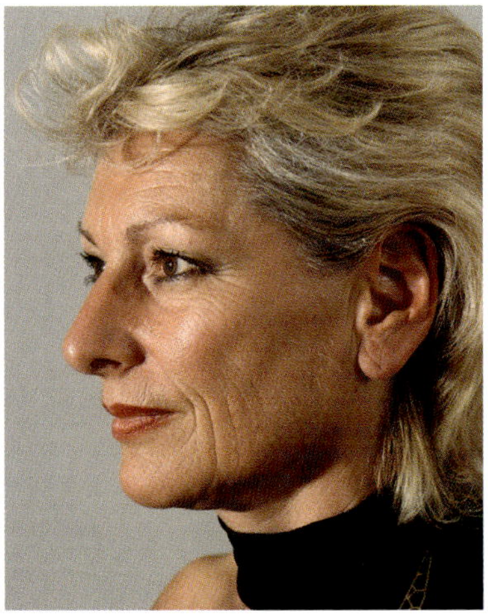

1b

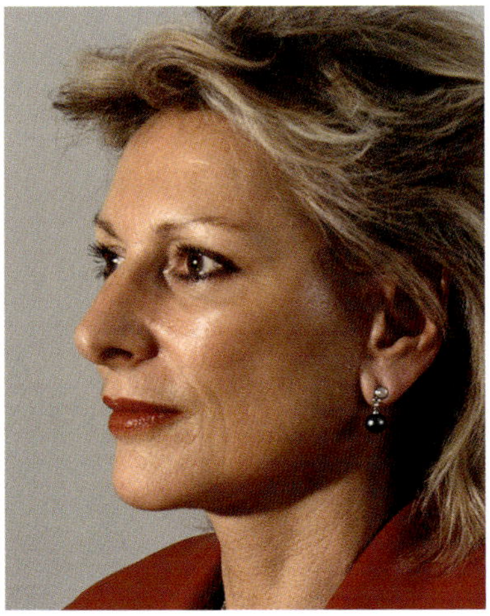

1c

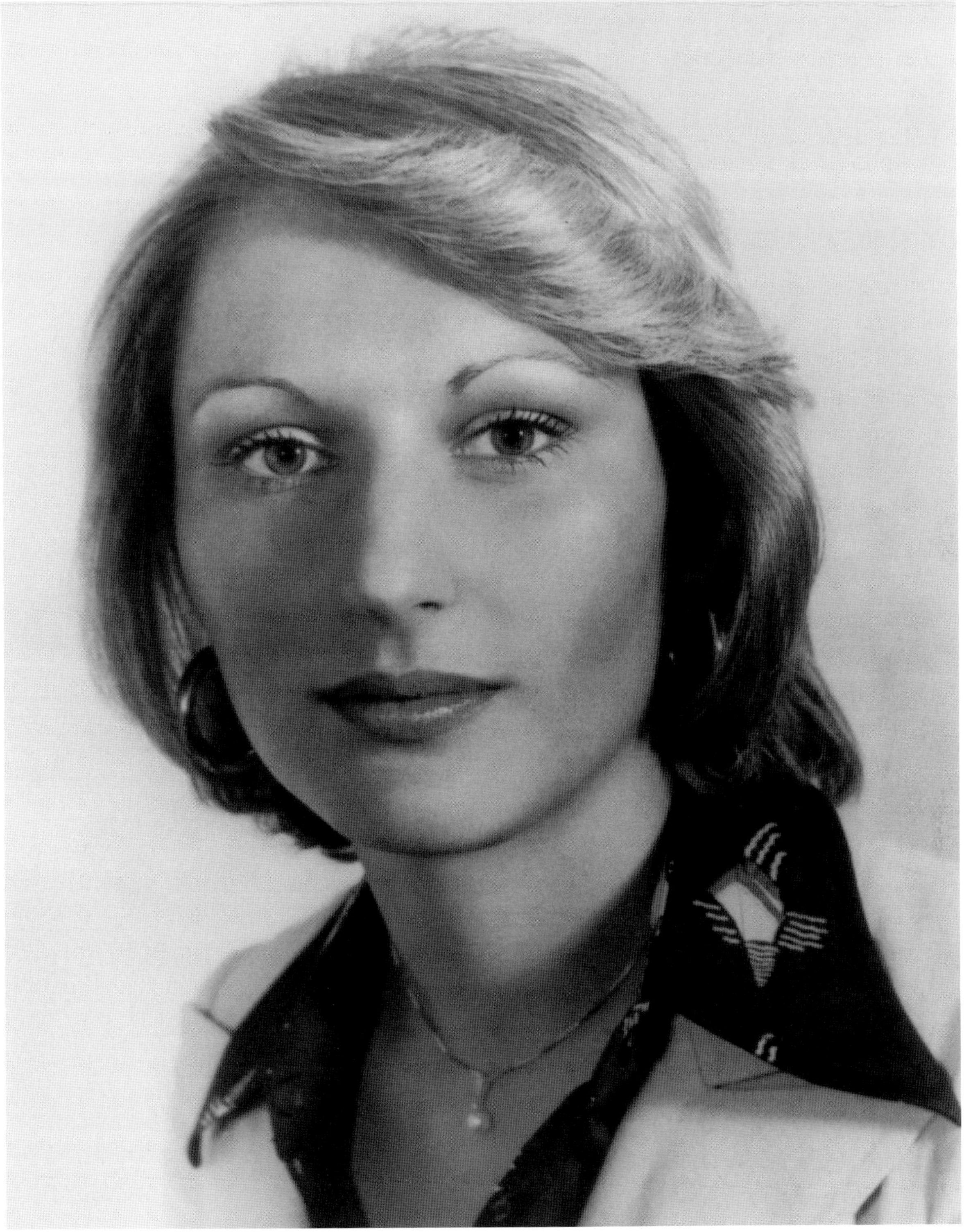

1d

1a Surgical sketches of the operating techniques

1b Before the operation

1c After face and neck lift with SMAS and platysmaplasty, micro liposculpture, upper and lower blepharoplasty, micro lipofilling of upper and lower lip, injections of Vistabel®(Botox®) in forehead region

1d Ideal of youthfulness

Nowadays many people elect to have rejuvenation surgery when they notice the first signs of ageing. Some people may become aware of and bothered by these changes in their late thirties but this occurs more commonly in their forties. Excellent results can be seen in younger patients because skin elasticity is usually very good. Even so, women and men in their fifties, sixties, seventies - and sometimes even older - can take great advantage of the benefits of aesthetic rejuvenation surgery, provided they are in excellent health. The next few pages describe the most common current plastic surgery techniques capable of counteracting the effects of facial ageing.

The passage of time inexorably leaves its traces upon the human body, in each organ and every body cell. The skin of the face ages more quickly and more evidently because it is exposed to the sun's rays and to a vast variety of subtle influences.

The ageing process of the skin is linked to the organism as a whole. It is an inexorable biological phenomenon. Nonetheless, this process differs from individual to individual because of many factors: the mental and physical health of the individual, heredity, style of life, various traumas, and so on.

The principal modifications of the skin over time are due to the loss of cutaneous elasticity and of muscular tone. There are distinct morphological changes in the skin. In the epiderm, cell division slows down, giving rise to slower tissue regeneration. Repeated exposure to the sun, as well as a reduction of cutaneous gland activity (sebaceous and sweat glands) cause a degree of dryness and a slightly scaly appearance of the skin. The collagen and elastin fibers have a diminishing amount of new collagen and elastin substance and tend to atrophy.

Gravitational force brings with it sagging of the skin and underlying tissues (downward migration). These alterations can also be accompanied by an increase in fat deposit tissue in the area of the cheeks, chin and neck. Apart from the wrinkles resulting from the sagging and the changes of the facial contours, smaller wrinkles appear where facial muscles contract - princi-

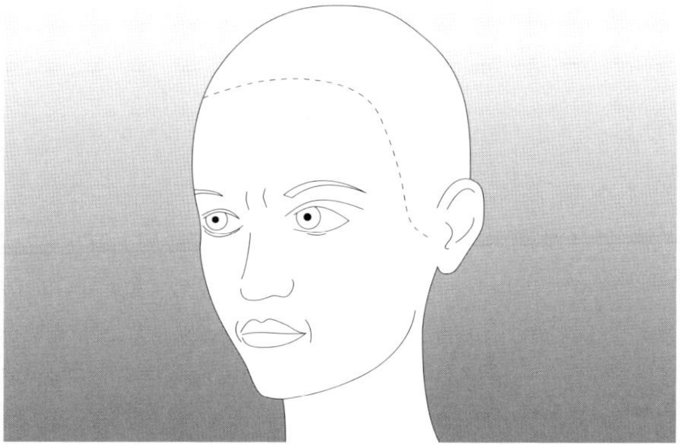

2

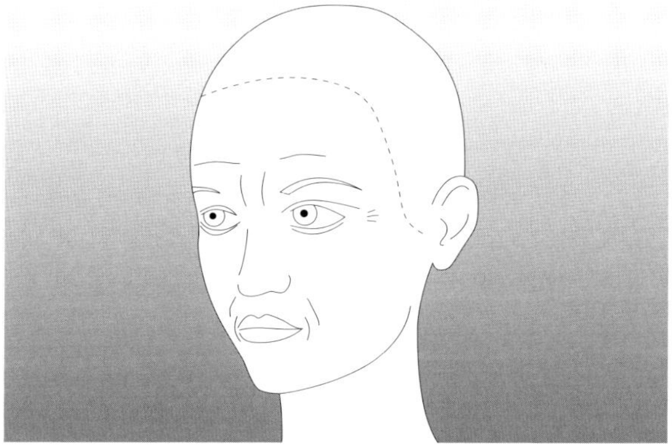

3

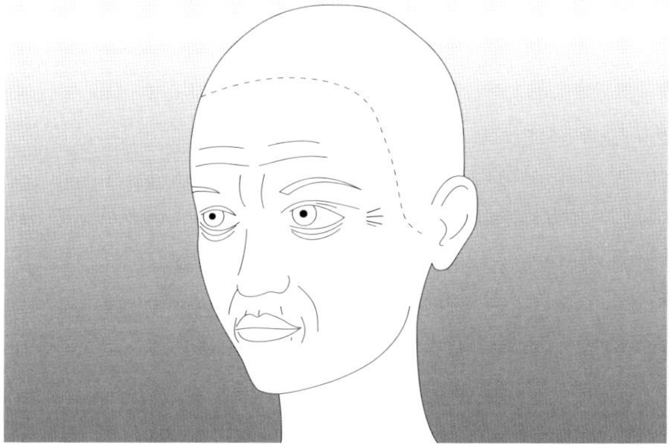

4

2–6 Age-related changes: 25–30 years, 30–40 years, 40–50 years, 50–60 years, 60–70 years

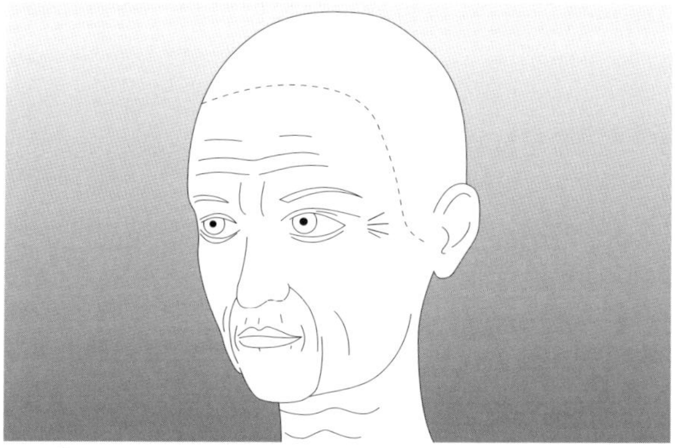

5

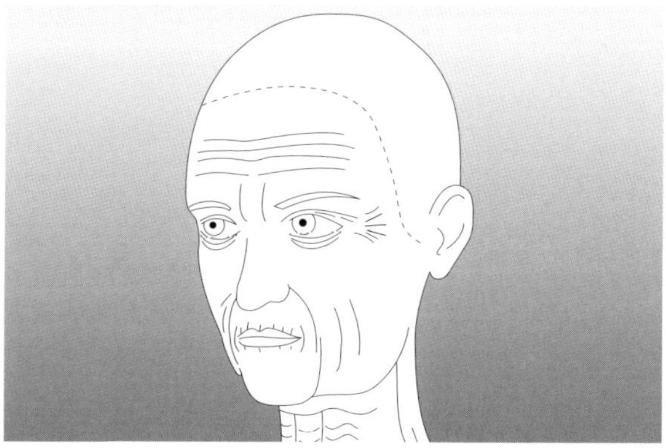

6

pally on the forehead, between the eyebrows on the outer side of the eyelids and around the mouth and the upper and lower lip.

The most noticeable changes of the skin appear generally first around the eyelids, then on the cheeks, in the neck and around the mouth. This process varies of course from one person to another and from one area of the face to another.

The nose undergoes certain changes of age as do other parts of the face. Usually a slight drooping and increased bulbousness of the tip occur (cf. the chapter on aesthetic rhinoplasty).

The age-related changes are illustrated in a very generalizd and simplified manner as follows (figs. 2–6):

25/30 years: Expression wrinkles appear between the eyebrows. Small, thin wrinkles become apparent on the lower eyelids and small creases tend to develop at the corners of the lips (fig. 2).

30/40 years: Horizontal wrinkles appear on the forehead and the wrinkles between the eyebrows are accentuated. The upper eyelids begin to droop slightly and small bags and wrinkles appear on the upper and lower eyelids. Crow's feet also begin to appear. The nasolabial folds become accentuated (fig. 3).

40/50 years: The horizontal wrinkles on the forehead and the frown lines are clearly visible. The crow's feet are deeper. The upper eyelids sag more and bags have increased. The bags of the lower eyelids are more accentuated and the fine wrinkles of the lower eyelids more visible. The nasolabial folds become deeper. Fine wrinkles may appear on the upper and lower lip and around the lips (fig. 4).

50/60 years: the forehead and eyebrows usually present a slight sagging and the creases of the forehead and between the eyebrows become deeper. In general, there is also distinct sagging in the area of the cheeks and in the neck and a deepening of the folds at the outer side of the mouth and at the root of the nose. The lips become somewhat thinner. The nasal tip often descends slightly. Deposits of fat can exist in the lower part of the cheeks and the neck region (fig. 5).

60/70 years: All the changes already mentioned are accentuated. The forehead and eyebrows drop further. The skin of the cheeks sags further and the platysma muscles of the neck region become more distended. The wrinkles on the upper and lower eyelids are more visibale, as are the crow's feet and the wrinkles in the forehead, in the face and neck, and the vertical lines on the upper and lower lips and the wrinkles at the corners of the lips (fig. 6).

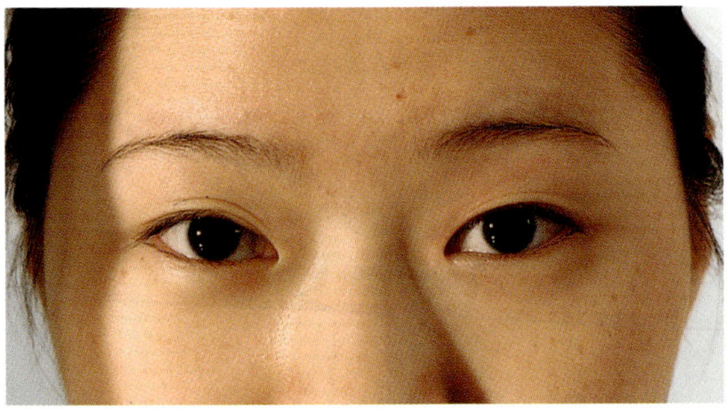

7a

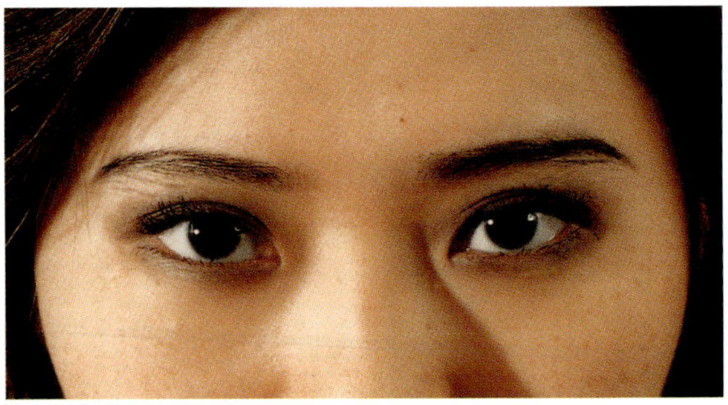

7b

Eyelid Surgery (Blepharoplasty)

The eyes are a focal point of the face and a prime element for youthfulness and beauty. Marked wrinkles, unsightly creases, bags and pouches on upper and lower eyelids are major contributing factors to the ageing face and can give the entire face a tired or sad expression. Drooping upper eyelids may even interfere with vision.

The aim of blepharoplasty is the removal of excess skin and the elimination of the wrinkles of the eyelids, as well as the bags (fat hernias). This intervention notably improves the expression of the eyes and produces a remarkable rejuvenation effect (figs. 7a,b, 8a,b 9a,b). It sometimes provides an increase in the field of vision and better resistance to eye fatigue.

Blepharoplasty is a small but delicate aesthetic intervention that requires great surgical finesse from the surgeon. It is one of the oldest procedures in the aesthetic surgery repertoire (see Pioneers of Aesthetic Facial Surgery).

The upper and lower eyelids can be operated at the same time or separately. Blepharoplasty is often performed together with a facelift, forehead and eyebrow lift or with any other rejuvenative procedures of the face.

Patients of Asian origin may choose a blepharoplasty to "enlarge" their eyes. Their eyelids do not have a fold and appear sometimes very large. The excess fat and skin are removed according to the conventional method, which is combined with a special technique to create an eyelid fold (fig. 9a,b)

In eyelid surgery there are no serious complications if the operation is performed by an experienced and qualified plastic surgeon. However small or insignificant the scar may be, it should not be forgotten that any surgical procedure leaves a trace. Scars due to blepharoplasty are usually invisible because the incisions are made in the natural skin creases. Postoperative infection and bleeding are extremely rare and easily treated.

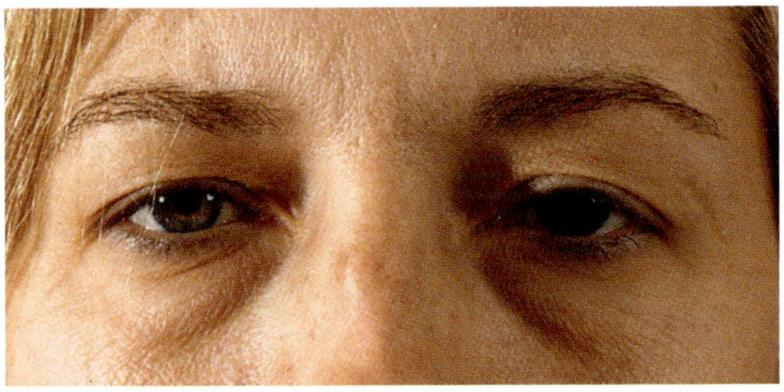

8a

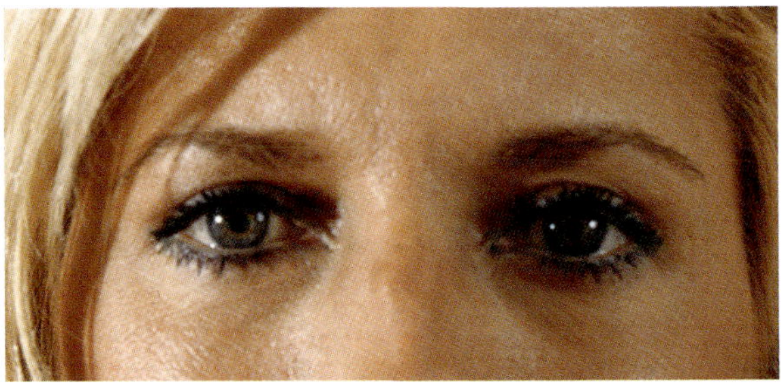

8b

7a,b Upper blepharoplasty, before and after

8a,b Upper and lower blepharoplasty, before and after

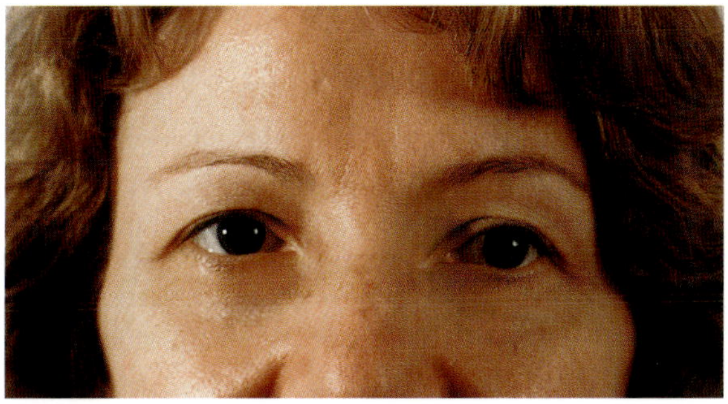

9a

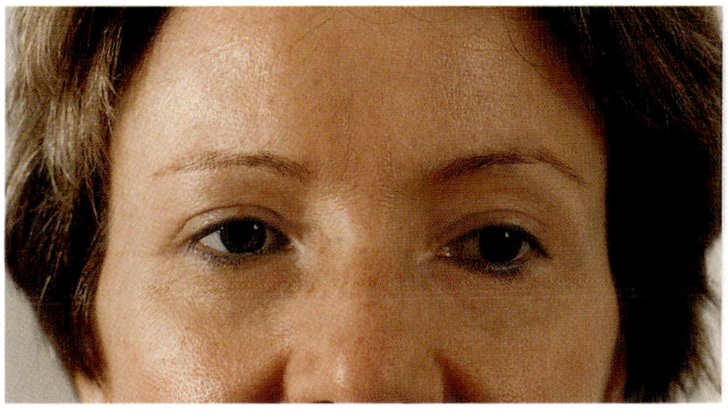

9b

Blepharoplasty is usually performed on an out-patient basis and always under local anaesthesia and sedation.

Operating technique

a) Upper eyelids

The skin to be excised is carefully measured and marked before the operation with the patient in a sitting position. The incisions are situated above and below the crease of the upper eyelid (fig. 10a). For minor corrections, the incision is two to three centimetres long: however, if there is a lot of excess skin at the outer corner of the eyelid, the incision can extend into the crow's feet area. The skin is detached and the excess is removed, usually together with a small muscular band. Through small supplementary incisions the surplus adipose tissue (fat hernias) is removed (fig. 10b). The wound is closed with fine sutures (fig. 10c). In general, an upper blepharoplasty requires half an hour to three quarters of an hour, depending upon the extent of surgery involved.

b) Lower eyelids

The amount of skin to be excised is also carefully measured and marked with the patient in a sitting position. The incision is made just below the edge of the lower eyelids in a natural line or crease (fig. 10a). The eyelid is undermined between the skin and the muscle or behind the muscle. Small supplementary incisions are made, if it is indicated to remove an adequate amount of the fatty tissue (fat hernias) (fig. 10b). Very often, instead of removing a part of the fat hernias, the deep tissue (septum orbitale) is tightened in order to reposition the fat hernias. After careful micro-coagulation, the wound is closed with fine sutures (fig.10c).

Some patients, particularly in the younger age group, have visible fat pockets on the lower eyelids without any excess skin. In this case, a trans-conjunctival blepharoplasty can be performed. With this technique, the incisions are made on the inside of the lower eyelids, from where the necessary amount of the fat pads is removed.

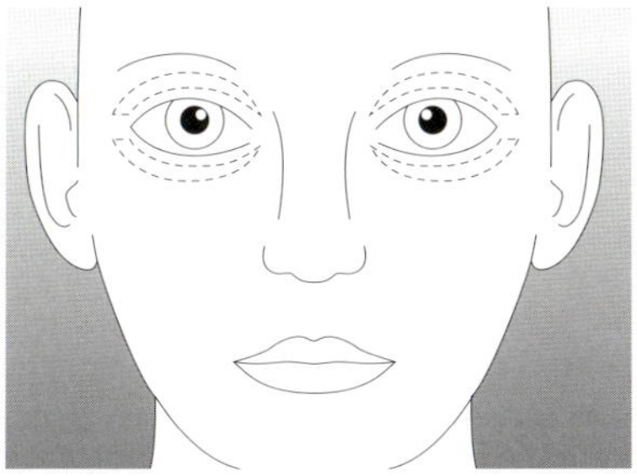

10a

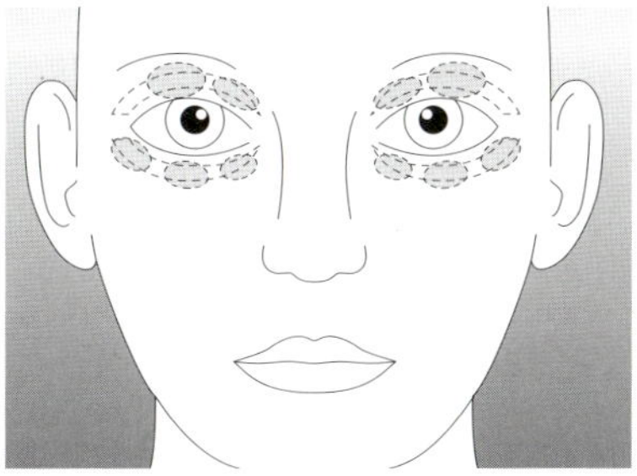

10b

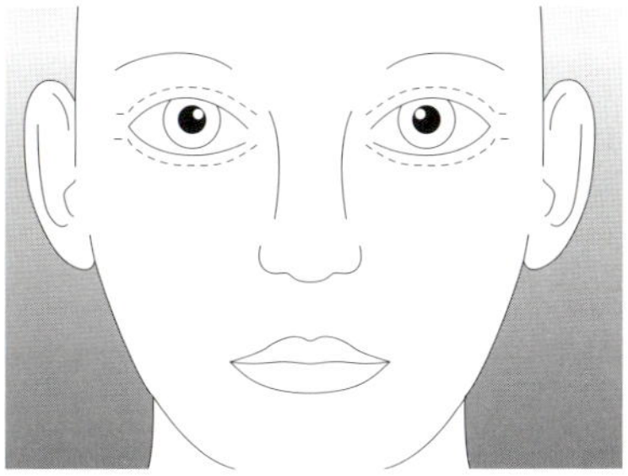

10c

9a,b Upper blepharoplasty, before and after
10a Incisions made in natural skin folds of the eyelids
10b Removal of excess skin, including fat pockets
10c Fine sutures of the incisions

The lower blepharoplasty lasts between half an hour and three quarters of an hour, depending on its scale.

Postoperative considerations

Swelling and bruises (ecchymoses) will appear around the eyes within twenty-four hours after the operation, but will gradually disappear within ten days. All sutures will be removed by the fourth or fifth day.

Strenuous exercises should be avoided during the first post-operative days. It is reassuring to know that make-up may be used three to five days after the operation to conceal any discoloration. Most patients will be able to resume a normal social life one week after surgery.

Important Elements

The region around the eyes contributes substantially to the overall facial appearance. To preserve the natural harmony of this expressive part of the face, blepharoplasty must be planned with extreme precision. It is essential to determine exactly the amount of skin and fat pads to be removed.

If the protuberance of the skin on the upper eyelid is caused mainly by sagging of the forehead and eyebrows, a blepharoplasty alone is not sufficient to obtain the desired effect. A forehead and eyebrow lift will ensure a natural and harmonious result, possibly in conjunction with a small upper blepharoplasty.

Forehead and Eyebrow Lift

The forehead and eyebrow lift is a relatively new surgical procedure that has evolved rapidly during the last twenty years. Since a few years it has often been performed by an endoscopic technique. The forehead and eyebrow lift allows all the wrinkles on the forehead to soften and even, in certain cases, removes them entirely. This lifting procedure permits the upward repositioning of the eyebrows as well. The space between the eyes and the eyebrows is increased, an important sign of beauty. This intervention can also considerably diminish the wrinkles known as crow's feet, a refinement which eyelid surgery alone cannot achieve. (figs. 11a,b, 12a,b).

One of the great advantages of the forehead lift is that it can prevent the reappearance of a number of expression wrinkles, especially the frown lines, by specifically altering some of the underlying muscles. This also helps to create a much longer-lasting result. To visualize the benefits of a forehead and eyebrow lift, the closed fingertips have to be placed on each side at the middle and outer part of the eyebrows and the skin has to be slid gently upwards and outwards to raise forehead and brows. This also allows one to see the extent to which wrinkles can be improved.

A notable sagging of the eyebrow arches is always associated with drooping upper eyelids and attendant wrinkles. In this instance an upper blepharoplasty will not permit good

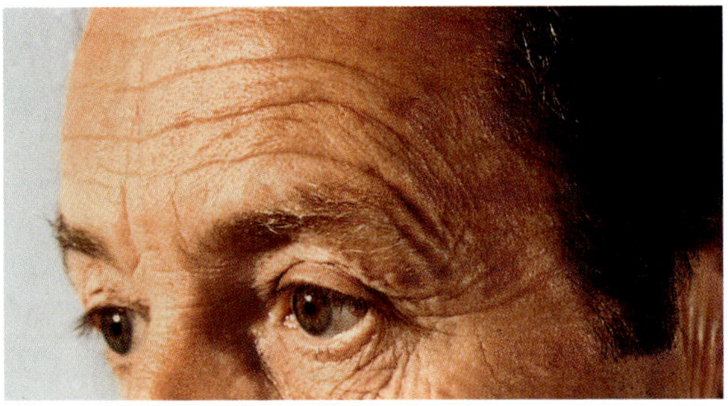

11a

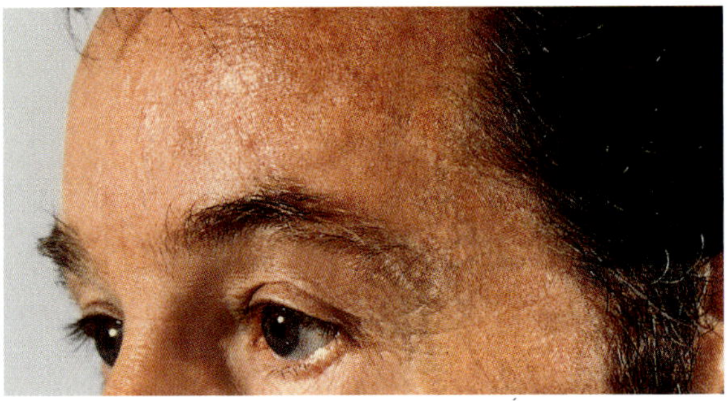

11b

11a,b Forehead and eyebrow lift, before and after

results aesthetically. A forehead and eyebrow lift would achieve the aesthetic results desired. A small blepharoplasty may be performed in conjuction with the forehead lift. Small wrinkles and furrows of the forehead are usually treated by dermabrasion, chemical peel or laser resurfacing (cf. Chapter on surface treatments or filling treatments). The forehead and eyebrow lift is often performed at the same time as a neck and facelift.

There is always a temporary diminution or loss of sensitivity in the operated skin area. Normal sensitivity gradually returns after a few months, although on rare occasions some numbness may persist. No injury can be caused to the small nerve controlling the movements of the eyebrow and forehead if the operation is performed by a qualified and experienced plastic surgeon. After this type of intervention, infections and post-operative hematomas are extremely rare and easily treated.

Forehead and eyebrow lifts are generally performed under local anaesthesia and sedation.

Surgical procedure

The conventional incision extends from ear to ear, behind the hairline (fig. 13a I). If the hairline is high or receding on the forehead, the incision may be placed just along the hairline to avoid adding even more height to the forehead (fig. 13a II). When the forehead lift is performed using endoscopy, several tiny incisions are made in the scalp. The placement of the incisions may vary (fig. 13a III). The skin and muscles of the forehead region are then carefully undermined so that the muscles of the forehead that cause specific wrinkles can be altered or released (fig. 13b). The excess skin is removed and the eyebrows are lifted to a more pleasing position according to the precise pre-operative measurement. The scalp incisions are closed with metal clips that provide maximum protection for the hair follicles and optimal scarring results.

The forehead and eyebrow lift is quite often performed by an endoscopic technique. The endoscope – a thin tube with a light at the end, attached to a micro video-camera that is connected to a video monitor – is inserted through one of the incisions, allowing the surgeon to have a clear view of the muscles and tissues beneath the skin.

With special endoscopic instruments that are inserted through another incision, the forehead skin and the muscles are lifted and the adequate amount of muscles removed to produce a smoother appearance of the forehead. The forehead and eyebrows are also lifted and secured in the higher position by special sutures or screws.

The endoscopic technique has the advantage of requiring minimal incisions, but it may not be equally beneficial for all patients, because in some cases it does not allow as much accuracy as the open technique.

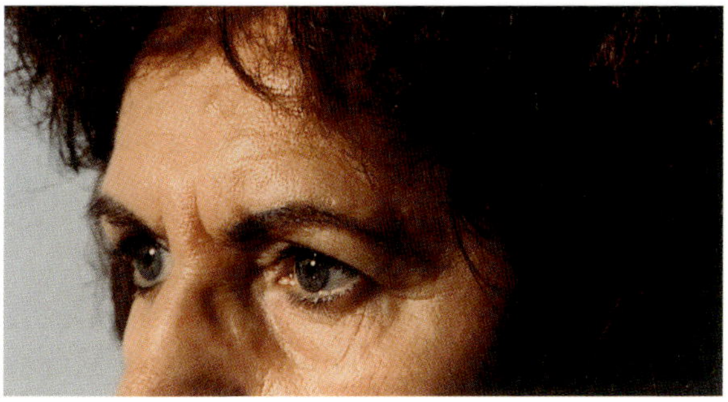

12a

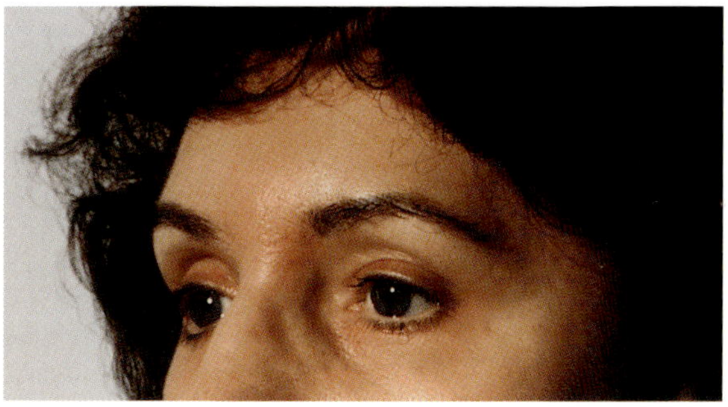

12b

12a,b Forehead and eyebrow lift, before and after

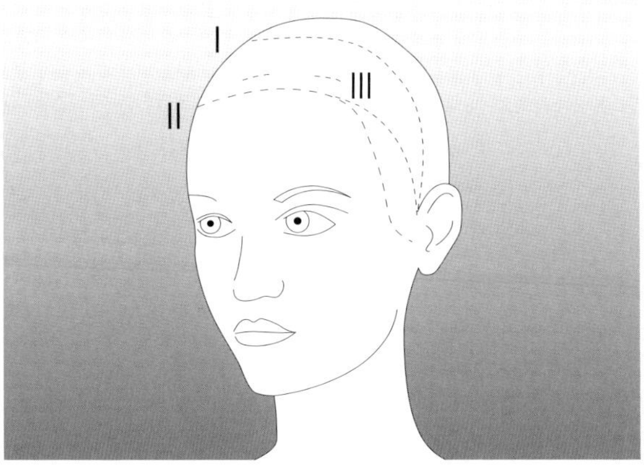

13a

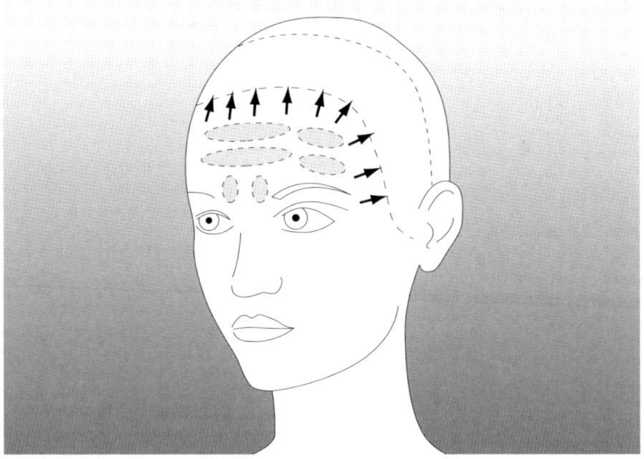

13b

In general, a forehead and brow lift lasts between sixty and ninety minutes, according to its scale.

Postoperative considerations

After this intervention, most patients spend a night under medical supervision. Some swelling and skin discoloration on the operated areas are natural and may involve the eyelid and upper cheek areas as well. The bruises disappear gradually within one to two weeks. Swelling is most evident the second day after surgery, thereafter diminishes considerably within the following days and will be almost totally resolved within two to three weeks. These postoperative manifestations vary considerably from one individual to another. All stitches or staples will be removed between ten days and two weeks following surgery. Strenuous exercises should be avoided during the first post-operative days. Most patients can resume a normal social life between seven and ten days after the operation.

Important elements

The detailed planning of a forehead and eyebrow lift must be preceded by a precise analysis and assessment of the patient's facial harmony. It is not only the static but also the dynamic anatomy of the face that is of importance.

Certain generalisations may be made about the aesthetically pleasing forehead and orbital region. A harmonious frontal and orbital region is ideally characterized by a relatively smooth forehead and well-positioned eyebrows. The position and shape of the eyebrows determine to a large extent the facial expression in the fronto-orbital region. An accurate diagnosis is therefore of fundamental importance, in this region of the face.

Eyebrows should be parallel to the orbital rim to give an attractive appearance and enhance the youthful character of a face. In the rest position, the outer end of the eyebrows should be approximately at the same height as, or slightly higher than the inner end. After a successful forehead and brow lift most wrinkles due to facial expressions, particularly lines between the eyebrows, hardly ever form again if they have been treated by an appropriate surgical technique involving muscle weakening by partial excision.

Every successful result of an aesthetic facial rejuvenation operation is based primarily on the harmonization of the overall facial expression. An aesthetic intervention in the frontal and orbital region therefore usually has to be combined with corresponding operating procedures in the central and lower parts of the face and in the neck region.

13a Incision for forehead lift a few centimetres from the hairline (I) On the hairline (II). Small incisions for forehead lift using endoscopy (III)

13b Removal of small parts of muscle, repositioning of the tissues

Face and Neck Lift

This surgical procedure improves the contours of the face and, especially, the deep wrinkles resulting from sagging of the skin and underlying tissues due to the ageing process. The lifting not only of the skin, but also of the deeper tissue layer in the face and of the superficial muscle in the neck is important. It improves far more the contour of the face, and particularly good results are obtained in the neck area and ensure a more lasting effect. The excess fatty tissue in the cheek and neck area is, if necessary, also removed (figs. 14a,b, 15a,b)

To visualize the potential effect of a face and neck lift, the middle fingers have to be placed on the cheek bones and thumbs on the lower jaw and the skin has to be drawn backwards and upwards.

A face lift however can contribute only slightly to the elimination of the small wrinkles surrounding the mouth, while it has no effect on the fine wrinkles located on the upper and lower lip. They result from muscular contractions and are etched on the skin itself. Dermabrasion, chemical peel or laser resurfacing are the indicated treatments, and they are usually employed as part of the face lift procedure. Certain fine wrinkles in this area may be treated effectively by injections of hyaluronic acid or collagen.

In order to ensure an optimal harmonious rejuvenation, the face and neck lift is often combined with eyelid surgery, micro-liposculpture, surface treatments, filling treatments and not infrequently with a forehead and eyebrow lift. When a face and neck lift is performed by a qualified and experienced aesthetic surgeon, complications are extremely rare and always minor.

However small or insignificant the resultant scar may be, surgery always leaves a trace. The healing of a surgical wound and an incision is a complex process; this process of healing cannot be the same for everyone, and so the appearance of scars cannot be the same for all patients. Very rarely, scars can, with the passage of time, thicken and enlarge despite the best suture technique because of a significant scarring reaction (hypertrophic scarring). Most face and neck lift scars are usually invisible because incisions are made in natural skin creases. The scars behind the ears may be slightly visible because of an occasional scar reaction, but these are easily hidden by the hair. Localised loss of cutaneous tissue is exceedingly rare. It is due to inadequate microcirculation in the specific skin area and occurs almost exclusively in smokers. The scar tissue is corrected by subsequent surgery. There is always a temporary diminution or loss of sensitivity in the operated skin area. Normal sensation returns gradually over a period of a few months. Exceptionally, very small branches of motor nerves may be affected by micro-coagulation (haemostasis), resulting in a temporary dysfunction of some mimic muscles. Permanent facial paralysis cannot occur if the intervention is performed by a qualified aesthetic surgeon who has adequate experience with this type of intervention. Post-operative bleeding and infection are very rare and easily controlled.

Most face and neck lifts are performed by experienced plastic surgeons under local anaesthesia, in conjunction with deep sedation.

Surgical procedures

The surgical procedures used in men and women are very similar. The choice of site for the incision is very important if the final appearance is to look natural. The incisions are designed to keep the resultant scars as inconspicuous as possible. The incision is usually made in the scalp in the area of the temple and descends in front of the ear in natural skin creases. It continues behind the ear and curves to the hairline of the neck and into the scalp (fig. 14a). Sometimes the incision is made along the hair-

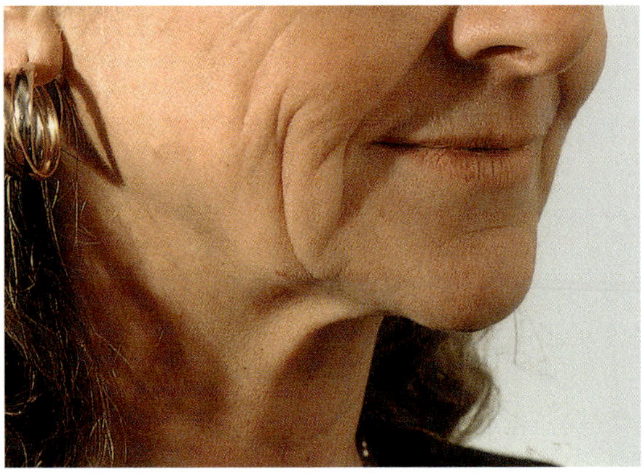

14a

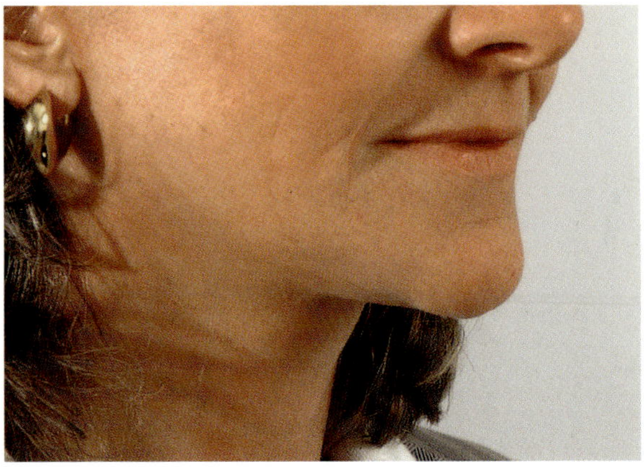

14b

line in the temple area; sometimes the incision is made inside the cartilage (tragus) in front of the ear. The aim is to ensure the least visible scars and a natural hairline with minimal displacement, and this requires surgical artistry. Depending upon circumstances, the skin of the temple region, the cheeks and the neck is detached from the underlying tissues to the extent necessary for the particular surgical technique selected and drawn upwards and backwards (fig. 14a). The excess skin is removed and the wound closed. However, a perfect aesthetic result is rarely achieved by skin undermining and skin resection alone. Supplementary corrections may be desirable and most often advisable.

For example, in the region of the cheeks, it is usually necessary to tighten deeper tissue layers, the SMAS (Superficial Musculo-Aponeurotic System, fig. 16b I), and in the neck the specific broad neck muscle, the platysma (fig. 16b II). When necessary, micro liposuction/liposculpture is used to remove excess adipose tissue at the lower cheek and jowl area, of the jaws and beneath the chin. This technique permits a considerable supplementary improvement of the natural contour of the face; the overall result is much more harmonious (fig. 16c). After suturing the deep layers (SMAS) and the neck muscle (platysma), the skin is re-draped, drawn upwards and backwards, and the excess excised as mentioned above. The skin is sutured in two layers, which ensures the best possible scarring result (fig. 16d). Metal staples are used to close the scalp incisions, ensuring maximum protection for the hair follicle.

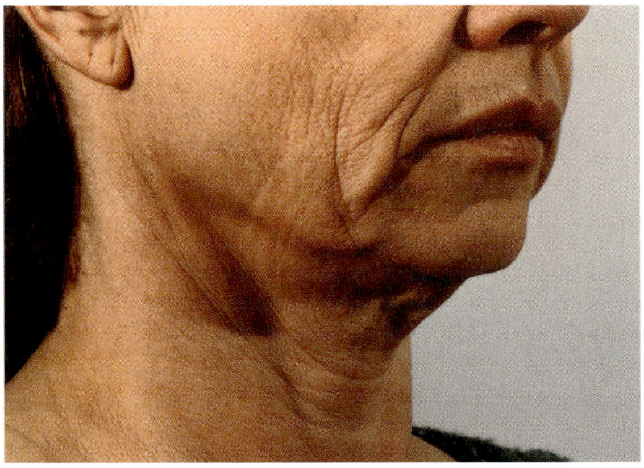

15a

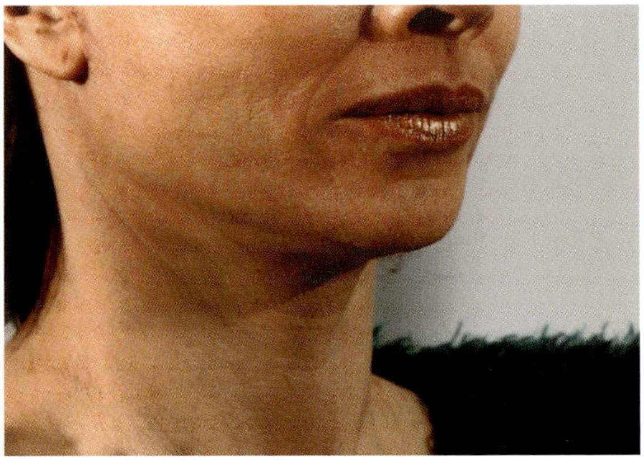

15b

14a,b Neck and face lift, before and after
15a,b Neck and face lift, before and after

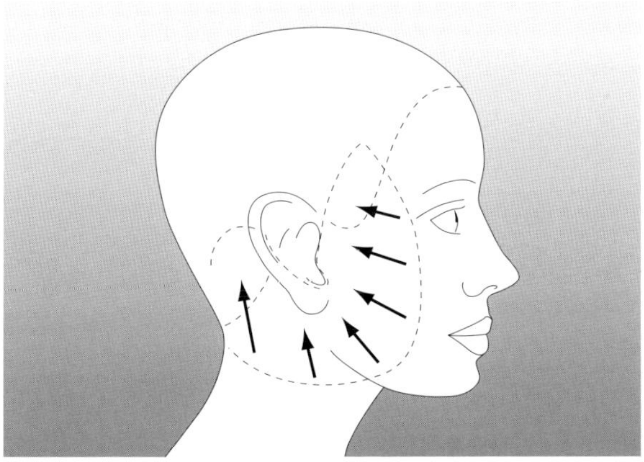

16a

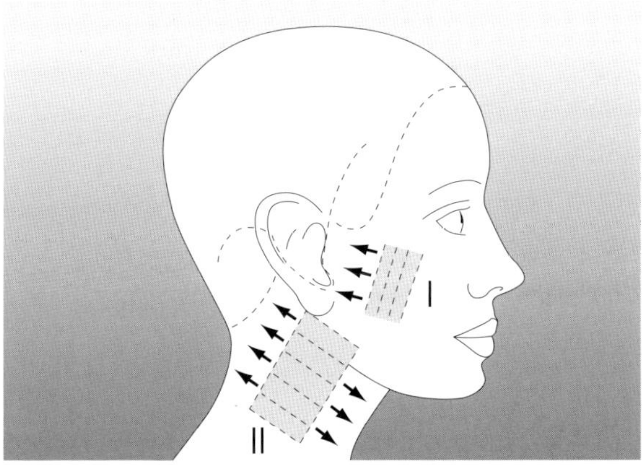

16b

On average, a face and neck lift procedure lasts from two to two-and-a-half hours, depending on its scale.

New surgical procedures are constantly being invented to solve the aesthetic problems presented by an ageing face. However, this does not necessarily mean that every new surgical procedure with a new designation ensures optimal results. Precaution is required before it has been tested and approved by qualified and reputed plastic surgeons.

Postoperative Considerations

There is usually no significant discomfort after surgery. Swelling and skin discoloration are common and will subside within a week or two. It is advised to elevate the head during rest periods; raising the head reduces the normal postoperative edema. The swelling is most evident the second day after surgery, thereafter diminishes rapidly within one to two weeks and disappears entirely within a few weeks (see chapter: Pre- and Postoperative Considerations pp. 104–107). These manifestations vary considerably from one individual to another.

Strenuous activities should be avoided during the first two to three weeks. It is possible to take up normal daily activities after the first postoperative days while observing these precautions. Unpleasant sensations and some numbness usually persist for several weeks, especially in the areas where the skin has been under-

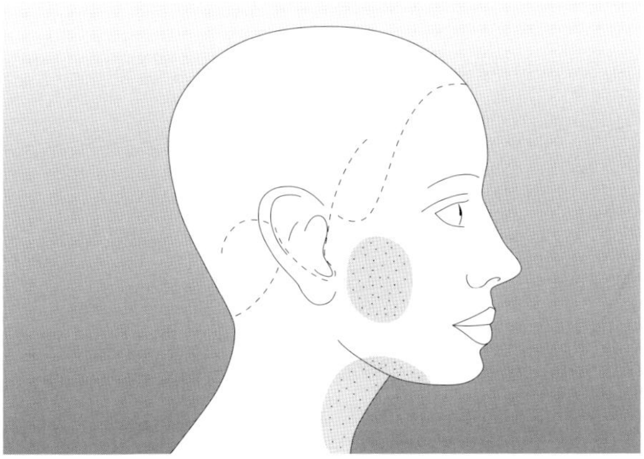

16c

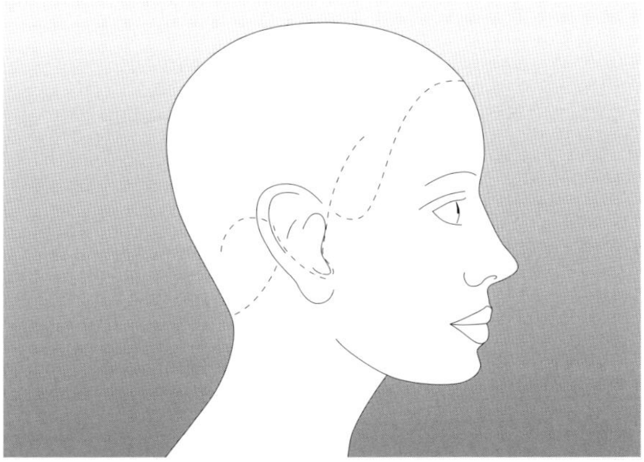

16d

16a Usual incisions for neck and face lift. Skin undermining, skin repositioning and removal of excess skin

16b Tightening of the deep tissue layers of the face (SMAS) (I) and/or of the superficial neck muscle (platysma) (II)

16c Removal of adipose tissue from the cheeks and neck, generally by micro liposculpture

16d Most of the scars are situated in natural skin folds and in the scalp mined. Special camouflage make-up may be applied to conceal any skin discolorations about one week after the operation. The stitches in front of the ear will be removed after about five days, the rest of the stitches and the staples within the following week. Most patients can resume their normal activities and be back to work about eight days to two weeks after surgery. Everything depends, of course, on the nature of the operation performed.

Important Elements

The face lift was long regarded as an operation intended primarily for fifty to sixty year-olds. Today, most of the patients are aged between fourty and fifty years. However, it's no longer exceptional to operate on patients in their late thirties, provided the indication is justified. Many of these younger patients seek the procedure in order to maintain their young appearance. Having a face lift at a younger age delays the need for more extensive surgery. Moreover, excellent results are also obtained well beyond sixty years. Everything depends on the patient's good physical health.

A successful rejuvenation effect also means taking account of multiple factors that generate the overall harmony of a person's face. Only proven surgical techniques should be used that are appropriate for the age-related alterations of the patient's face.

Face and neck lifts often afford a rejuvenation of eight to ten years, sometimes even fifteen, although of course the process of ageing always continues. But later the face looks much younger than without a face lift. The intervention genuinely slows down the process of tissue distension. Certain patients may wish to undergo a second surgical intervention, that is usually minor, ten to fifteen years later (cf. mini face lift), but the rules of harmony and naturalness have to be strictly observed and respected.

Mini Face Lift (Minimal Incision Face Lift)

The mini face lift or minimal incision face lift corrects sagging of the skin and the underlying tissues in the face and upper neck (fig. 17a,b). This type of face lift has the primary advantage of avoiding retro-auricular scars and of preserving the post-auricular hairline. There is less significant skin undermining in the region of the lower face and neck, and as a consequence less invasiveness than with the traditional face and neck lift (fig. 18a,b).

Except in patients with very minimal signs of ageing, the Superficial Musculo-Aponeurotic System (SMAS) in the face, and the superficial platelike muscle in the neck (platysma), have usually also to be elevated and repositioned in order to obtain the best possible result (fig. 18b I/II). The micro liposculpture technique, often used to remove deposited fat tissue in the lower jowl area and in the neck area, ensures a further harmonization of the contour of the face.

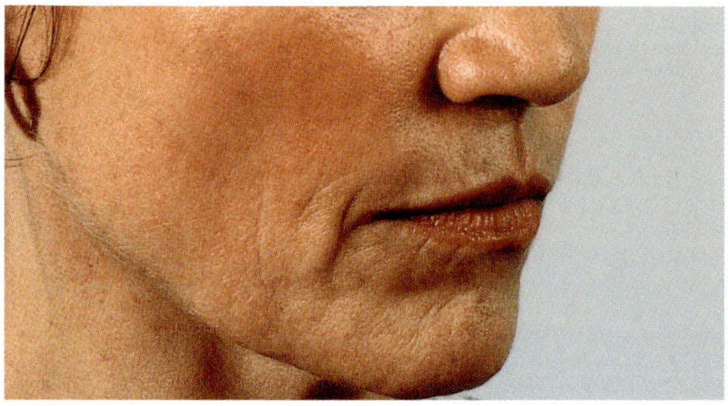

17a

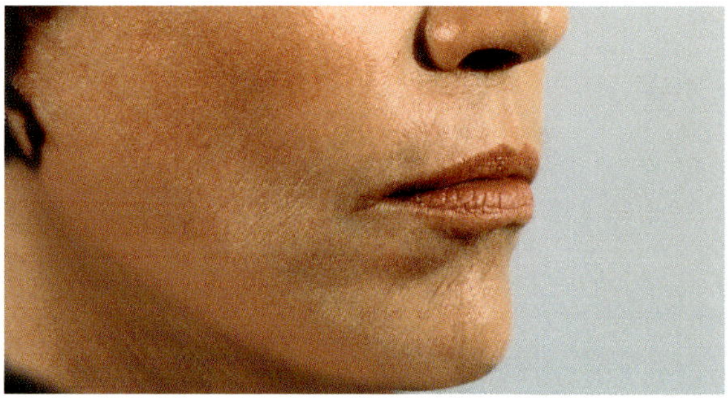

17b

17a,b Mini facelift, before and after

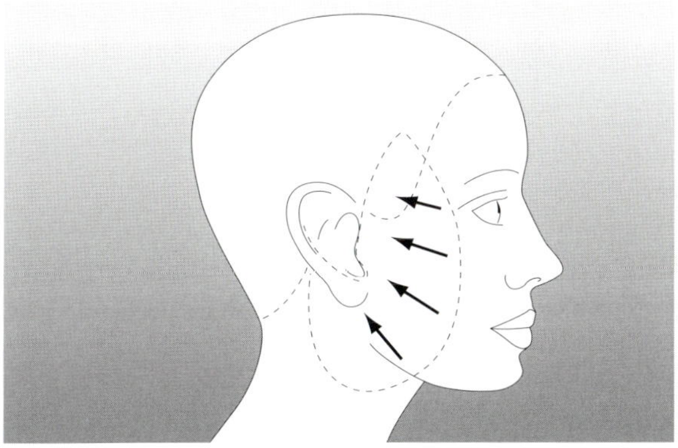

18a

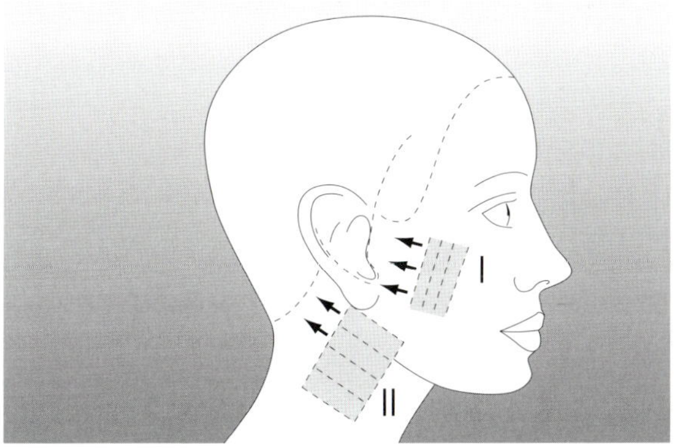

18b

This less traumatizing technique is very appropriate to correct the earliest signs of ageing. It is particularly indicated for younger, thirty-five to fourty-five year old patients and also for many older patients with moderate skin laxity in the lower cheek and cervical area. It is particularly suitable for patients that desire a second face lift – perhaps eight to ten years after their first procedure because they present usually quite moderate sagging of the skin.

A typical intervention lasts, between one and a half and two hours.

Important Elements
The mini facelift is an interesting alternative to the classical face and neck lift for many patients. It is less invasive and nevertheless offers excellent correction of the nasolabial folds, the laxity in the lower cheek region and submental region. It also permits a more rapid post-operative recovery, so that most patients can resume their normal social activities between seven to ten days after surgery. This technique however is not indicated for patients with severe cervicofacial skin laxity and important loss of skin elasticity. They benefit much more from a classical face and neck lift with a retro-auricular incision.

Micro Liposuction/Liposculpture

Micro liposuction/liposculpture has become a very common surgical procedure to remove localized deposits of fat from different parts of the face and neck in order to improve the contours of the face.

The development of these operating techniques a few years after the invention of liposuction and liposculpture have given new perspectives to aesthetic rejuvenation surgery (fig. 19a,b).

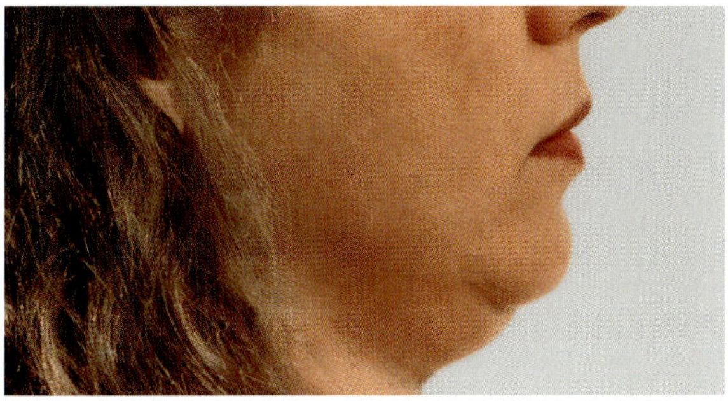

19a

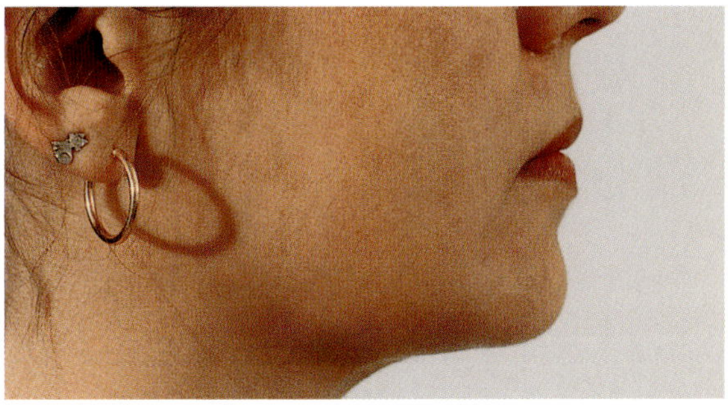

19b

18a Mini-facelift: incision on the temple and in front of the ear without a scar beyond the crease behind the ear. Skin undermining in the regions indicated, in the face and upper neck, skin repositioning and removal of excess skin
18b Tightening of the deep tissues of the face (SMAS) (I) and of the superficial muscle in the neck (platysma) (II)
19a,b Micro liposculpture, before and after

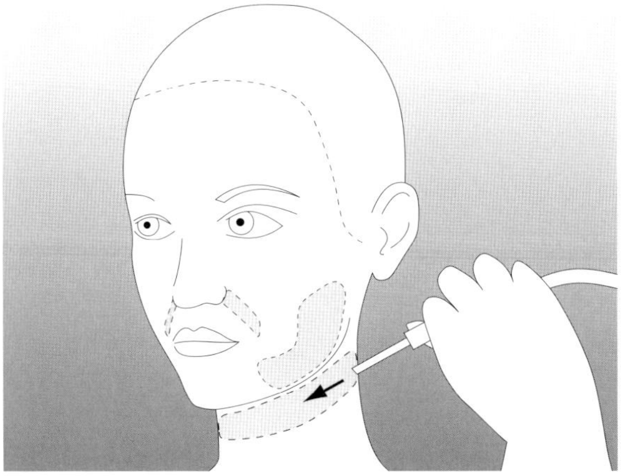

20

The technique is particularly well-suited to remove small deposits of fat from the lower cheek area, the neck and under the chin, provided the skin elasticity is good and tightens again properly after the intervention. Micro liposuction can improve the contours of the face and neck considerably (fig. 20).

Micro liposuction is often used alone, but it is also very commonly performed in conjunction with a face and neck lift to re-contour the lower face and neck and to enhance proper skin redraping (see Chapter: The Quest for Perfection in Facial Rejuvenation). The micro liposuction technique is performed with 2–2.5mm thick micro cannulas that are connected to a high pressure vacuum unit, and the micro liposculpture technique with cannulas of the same shape and same thickness, but connected to a special syringe that creates the vacuum.

Micro liposuction or micro liposculpture is generally performed under local anaesthesia in conjunction with deep sedation and on an outpatient basis

Surgical procedure

Before the operation, the surgeon marks precisely the skin to demarcate accurately the areas of aspiration and the location of very fine incisions, not exceeding 2 to 3 mm, behind the earlobes and under the chin. The small tubular cannulas are inserted through the incisions. Different, specific cannulas are used, connected to a high-pressure aspirator or a syringe. The cannulas are manipulated quickly in a fan-shaped manner so that numerous tiny micro-cylinders of adipose tissue are removed.

A typical operation requires fifteen to thirty minutes, depending on its scale.

Considerable swelling and some skin discoloration are usual in the treated areas. The discoloration disappears within one or two weeks. The swelling subsides completely only within one to two months, but will not be noticeable after ten days to two weeks. The special compression bandage, which it is advised to wear at night for two weeks, and lymphatic drainages will help to speed re-absorption of postoperative edema. It is usually possible to be back to social life three to five days after surgery.

Important Elements

Micro liposuction or micro liposculpture sometimes manages to produce some quite spectacular rejuvenation effects due to the good tissue retraction caused by the multiple "tunnelling" of the adipose tissue. An excellent command of the technique is however mandatory to obtain optimal results.

Surface Treatments

These methods are indicated to correct small skin irregularities, soften fine wrinkles and refinish scarred or blemished facial skin. General skin texture also becomes smoother and firmer (figs. 21a,b, 22a,b).

These procedures are by no means a substitute for a face and neck lift or a forehead lift, but they are often performed in conjunction with these rejuvenative surgical procedures.

20 Micro liposuction/liposculpture: cheeks, jaws, chin, neck,

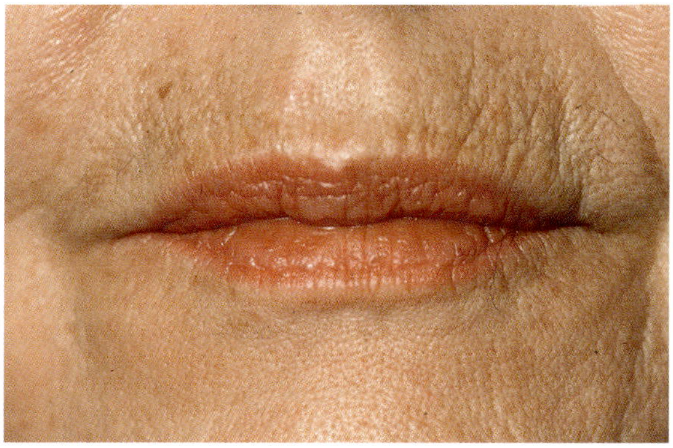

21a

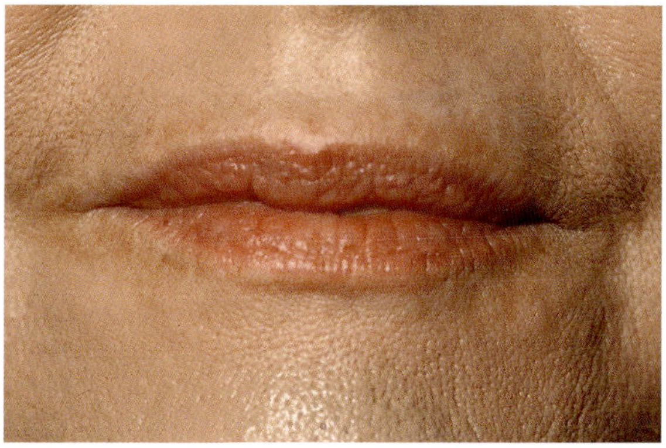

21b

All these methods can be used on the whole of the face, or only on some specific parts, such as the forehead, eyelids and upper or lower lips. For most patients the results are long-lasting.

In general, these interventions require between fifteen minutes and one hour, depending on the surface area to be treated and the technique used.

If these procedures are not done in conjunction with facial surgery, they are usually performed on an outpatient basis. Dermabrasion and laser resurfacing are performed under local anaesthesia with sedation and chemical peeling usually under sedation alone.

Chemical Peeling consists of applying a chemical solution (such as, for example, phenol, trichloroacetic acid, etc.) to different parts of the face or the whole face; the degree of penetration depends on the type of peel, the concentration of the solution and the quantity used (figs. 21a,b, 23a I / II). Chemical peeling is indicated to minimize the effects of ageing, such as fine lines and wrinkling and sometimes to remove certain skin blemishes associated with pigmentation problems.

Dermabrasion is carried out by a burr containing diamond particles, attached to a high-speed electrically operated instrument. Dermabrasion is normally used to erase fine wrinkles, but is also often employed to soften certain skin irregularities, such as tiny scars or acne scars. It is the most widely used technique for attenuating the fine wrinkles on the upper and sometimes on the lower lip, often in conjunction with a face and neck lift (figs. 22a,b, 23b I / II).

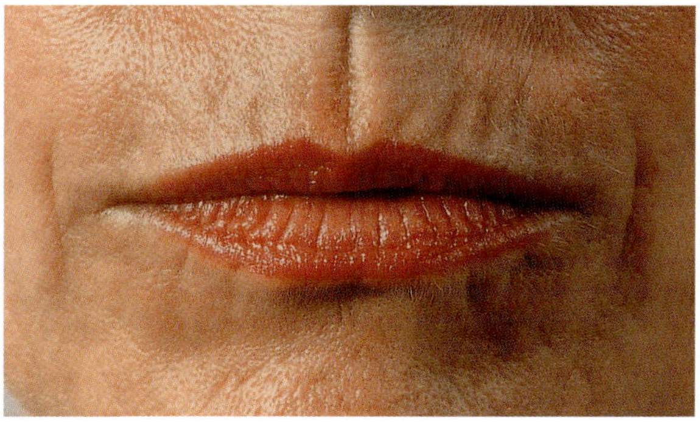

22a

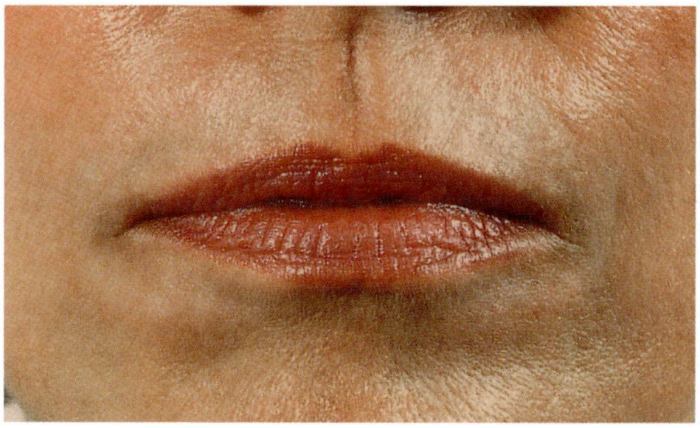

22b

21a,b Chemical peel, before and after

22a,b Dermabrasion, before and after

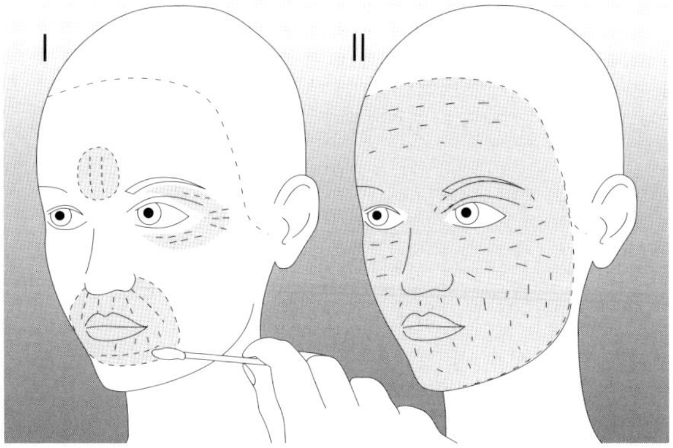

23a

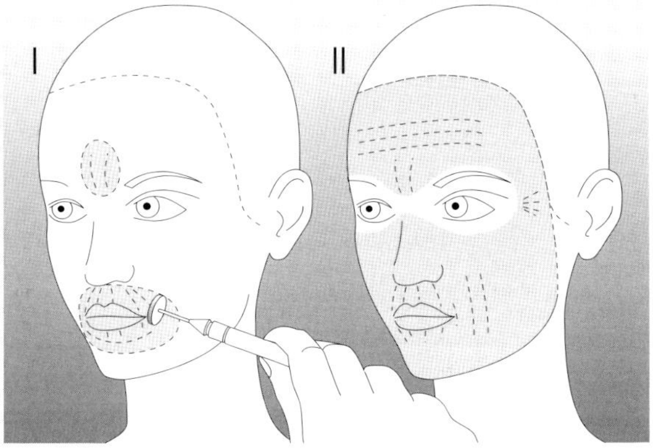

23b

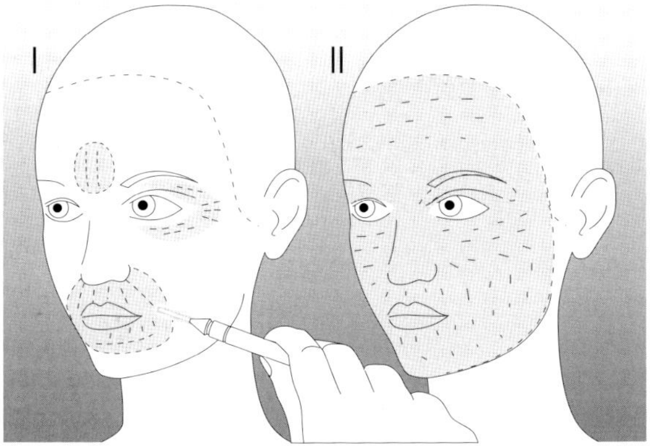

23c

Laser Skin Resurfacing is the most recent technique. The ultra-pulse laser is a computerized surgical laser system that delivers very high energy pulses of light. This procedure allows clean, precise, layer-by-layer removal of skin. This treatment has the same indications as dermabrasion and chemical peel (figs. 23c I / II).

All these techniques remove the upper layer of the skin. The resulting scab or crust will fall simultaneously with the formation of new skin. The surface wound heals within five to ten days depending on the depth and type of treatment. The surfaces treated will remain swollen for several days and the skin retains a reddish colour for a month or two, but rarely longer. As soon as the skin has healed, non-allergenic camouflage make-up may be applied. It is essential to use a sun block and to avoid all exposure until the reddish colour of the skin has completely faded.

Important Elements

Similar results can be obtained with the different methods. however, it is important to choose the appropriate procedure for the specific needs. Although these cosmetic procedures are a priori surface treatments, they are quite delicate and require a lot of expertise and know-how. A small error of judgement in relation to the depth of treatment can cause irreversible skin damage and as a consequence hypo- or hyperpigmentation, or even permanent scars. However, if these procedures are performed by a qualified and experienced specialist, they are effective and safe.

Botulinum Toxin

Botulinum toxin type A has been used for more than twenty years, especially in neurology and neuro-ophthalmology, to treat strabismus and a variety of neuromuscular disorders related to muscle hypertonicity and spasticity. Since 1992 botulinum toxin has been used in aesthetic medicine to weaken certain muscles related to expression lines, particularly in the upper part of the face, between the eyebrows, on the forehead and in the region of the crow's feet. Excellent results are also obtained by the treatment of wrinkles in the perioral area and the area of

23a Chemical peel in well defined regions (I) of the whole face (II)

23b Dermabrasion; labial folds and frown lines (I) of the whole face (II)

23c Skin resurfaced by ultrapulse laser: in specific regions (I) of the whole face (II)

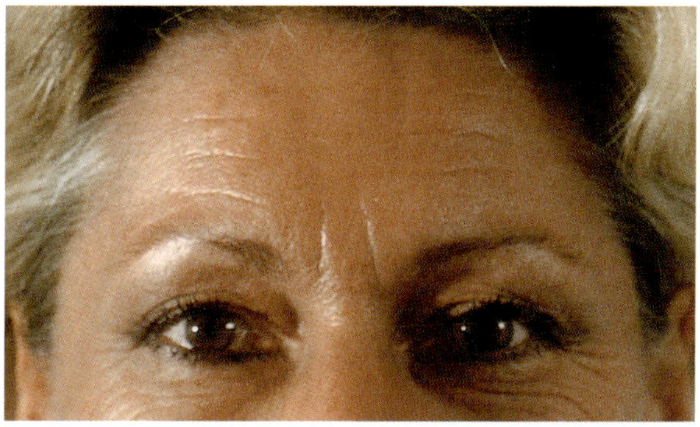

24a

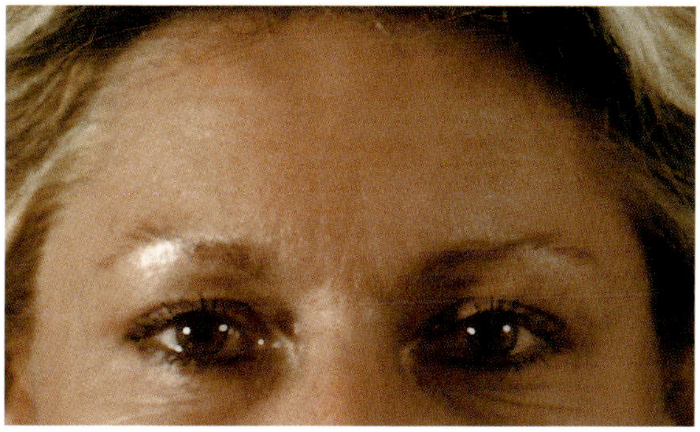

24b

the chin and of the hypertrophic vertical platysma muscle bands in the neck (figs. 24a,b, 25).

Type A botulinum toxin, produced by the Bacterium Clostidium botulinum, it exerts its effect at the neuromuscular junction by inhibiting the release of the nerve transmitter substance Acetylcholin. Type A botulinum toxin is actually the most potent of these toxins and has a particularly long duration of action. The American botulinum toxin, a purified neurotoxin complex of botulinum toxin type A, known as Vistabel®, or Botox®, is the most widely used. The toxin is injected by means of a very fine needle directly into the muscles responsible for the expression lines. The precise location of the injection points is of primary importance.

The positive aesthetic effects can be seen within three to five days after the injections and last on average between five and eight months without any change, then fade within a few weeks.

Normal activities can be resumed immediately after the injections. In rare cases patients experience a slight temporary bruising at the injection site. This can be easily covered by make-up. Very rarely the toxin may cause a temporary weakness in an adjacent muscle due to dissemination of the product. Such a complication is manifested by drooping of an eyebrow or eyelid, or by another form of facial asymmetry, but the effects of these injections are reversible.

However, if the treatment is performed by a specialist, who restricts the injections to carefully located sites, the incidence of these temporary side effects can be completely avoided. Very rarely a week after the original injections, a second small "touch-up" in a certain area might be necessary.

Important Elements

Although botulinum toxin injections do effectively soften expressional wrinkles, they cannot improve wrinkles caused by skin sagging or loss of skin elasticity, and cannot under any circumstances be a substitute for a forehead or face lift.

In the fronto-orbital region this technique produces spectacular results on the forehead creases, frown lines and crow's feet, particularly for patients who have little or no sagging in

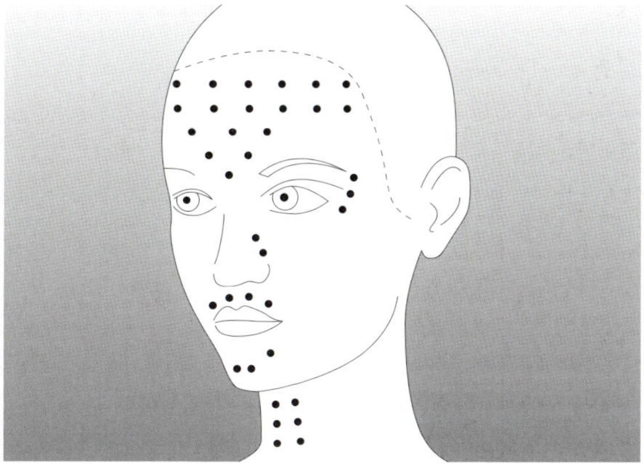

25

24a,b Injections of Botulinum toxin, fronto-orbital region, before and after

25 Usual injection points for botulinum toxin

this region. If the injections are done skilfully and precisely, a minor lifting effect with a slight eyebrow elevation can often be achieved comparable to that of a minor forehead and eyebrow lift. On the other hand, if there is significant sagging in the forehead region, only a surgical lift will produce the desired rejuvenation effect.

Filling Treatments

While very small surface wrinkles are best treated by chemical peels, dermabrasion or laser skin resurfacing, the injectable products are used to fill deeper lines and wrinkles, such as frown lines, nasolabial folds and wrinkles around the mouth, to fill up sunken areas of the face and to increase the volume of the lips.

Deep frown lines, deep horizontal lines on the forehead and deep wrinkles in the face, caused by excessive muscle activity or sagging skin, may be more effectively treated by aesthetic surgery, such as a forehead and brow lift or a face and neck lift.

Injectable products such as hyaluronic acid or collagen in different concentrations are substances that are routinely used to treat wrinkles in the forehead, crow's feet, nasolabial folds, wrinkles in the area of the cheeks and on the upper und lower lip and to enhance the volume of the lips.

Hyaluronic acid, produced by biotechnology, reveals several advantages in comparison with other injectable biomaterials. Hyaluronic acid is a natural polysaccharide polymer, which exists in identical form in the dermal layers of the skin. Hyaluronic acid is responsible for hydration of the dermis because of its water-binding capacities. Its concentration in the skin decreases with age. Due to an extremely effective stabilization method it was possible to obtain a formulation of hyaluronic acid that has a much longer residence time and stays in the skin usually more than a year, while remaining completely biocompatible and biodegradable.

The duration of the hyaluronic injections varies significantly from patient to patient. Usually the injections are repeated after six months to one year to maintain the result. (figs. 27a,b, 28).

Micro lipofilling is used primarily to fill deep wrinkles such as frown lines and nasolabial folds and to treat depressions in the face that are congenital or result from atrophy of the adipose tissue and to increase the volume of the lips. Micro lipofilling is commonly used today for contour augmentation of the face, for instance in the malar and cheek region (figs. 26a,b, 29).

Micro fat grafts are removed by means of a special small cannula and a syringe that creates a vacuum. After separating the solid from the liquid part, the resultant solid, ideal for trans-

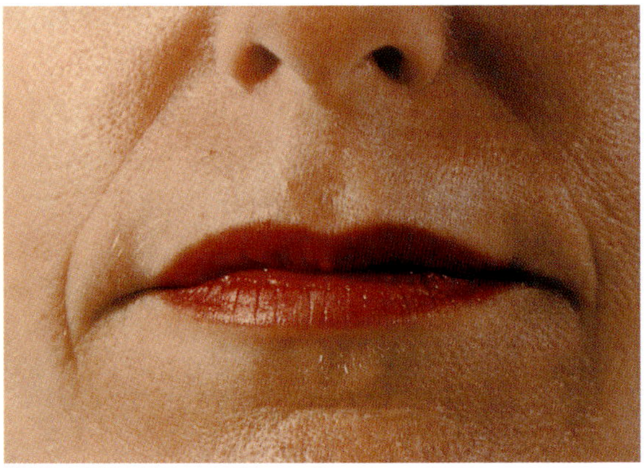

26a

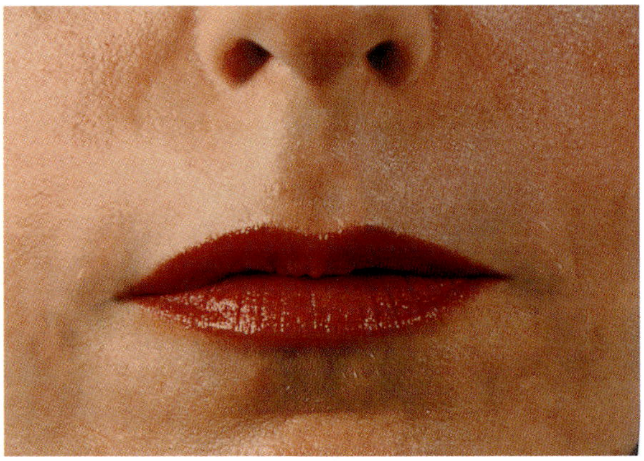

26b

26a,b Micro lipofilling of nasolabial folds and lips, before and after

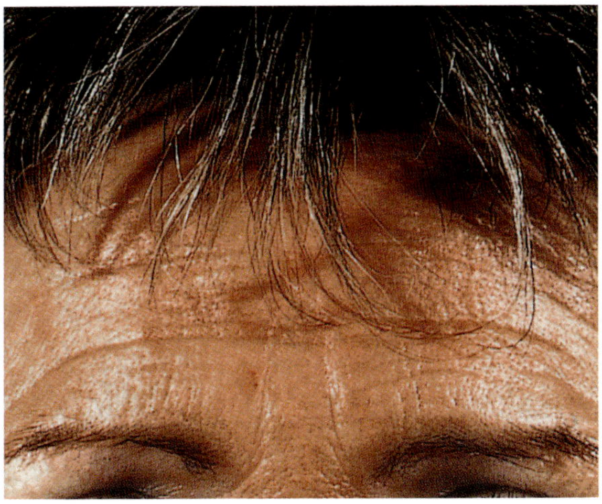

27a

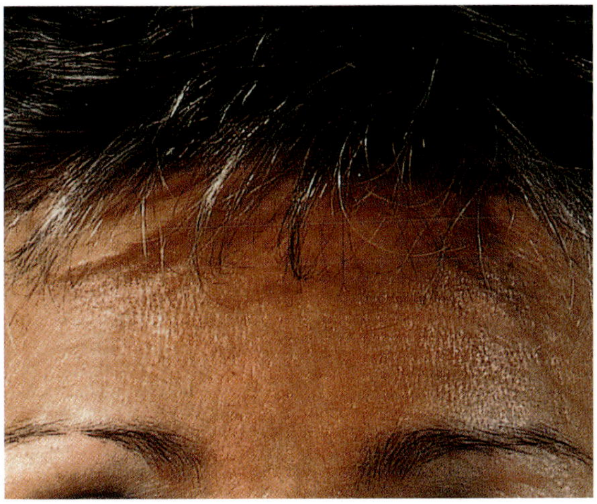

27b

plantation, is re-injected in the desired areas. The "donor" region may be at different points of the body, such as the inner side of the knees or the face in the case of facial micro liposculpture. Micro lipofilling is usually performed under local anaesthesia and sedation.

There is usually some swelling and bruising in the donor and recipient sites for a few days. A moderate swelling may last several weeks, especially if a large area has been filled.

The assimilation rate of the injected micro fat grafts varies from patient to patient. It depends on the location of the recipient site, the quality of tissue in this area, the quality of the transplanted micro fat grafts and many other factors. It is therefore often necessary to repeat the procedure during the next six to twelve months. However, many excellent and lasting results have been observed after only one or two injections.

Important Elements

Injectable products that are totally or partially non-degradable and stay in the body for an indefinite length of time have been shown to be undesirable. Such substances can cause chronic inflammatory reactions and indurations, sometimes even several years later. It is therefore advantageous to use only totally degradable materials.

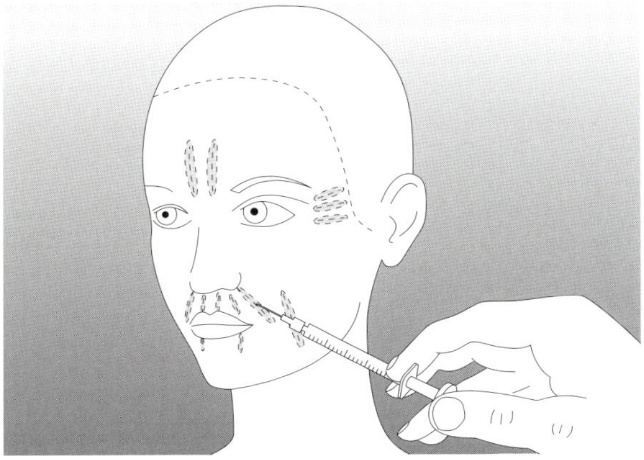

28

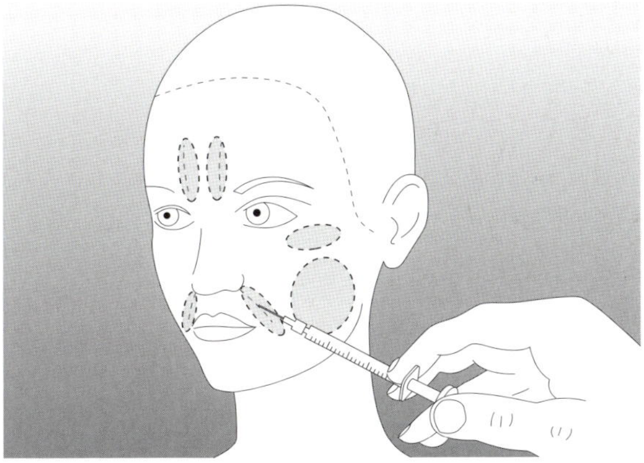

29

27a, b Injections of hyaluronic acid in frown lines and forehead wrinkles, before and after

28 Injectable products (e.g. hyaluronic acid) for frown lines, nasolabial folds, perioral wrinkles, crow's feet

29 Micro lipofilling for frown lines and nasolabial folds, deep wrinkles and depressions

Aesthetic Rhinoplasty

Aesthetic rhinoplasty is a surgical procedure used to reduce the size of the nose, to reshape the tip or the base of the nose, to remove a hump and/or to change the angle between the lower edge of the nose and the upper lip (figs. 30a,b). These changes are obtained by removing, shifting, or altering underlying bone and cartilage structures. Sometimes it is necessary to add tissue, usually cartilage, to obtain the desired shape. Depending on the particular case, the surgeon employs one or other of these operating techniques, either in isolation or in combination. Aesthetic rhinoplasty can also be combined with a therapeutic intervention of the nasal septum to relieve breathing problems.

The earliest recommended age for aesthetic rhinoplasty is between fourteen and sixteen, when the nose has attained nearly its fully-grown size; the operation may be performed at any subsequent age.

As a result of the ageing process the nose may become longer and the tip may droop slightly and become more bulbous. Often a small procedure to elevate and refine the tip of the nose will contribute greatly to a younger appearance of the face. Such a procedure is quite commonly performed together with face and neck lift surgery.

Small contour irregularity may occur following surgery, even if the surgeon has performed the operation with the greatest care. Additional minor surgery to ensure optimal results may exceptionally be required.

Aesthetic rhinoplasty is usually performed under local anaesthesia and sedation and on an outpatient basis.

Surgical procedure

Aesthetic rhinoplasty usually starts with internal incisions in the vestibulum of the nose (figs. 31, 32a). Sometimes, however, it is necessary to make a small external incision in the middle of the base of the nose (columella; fig. 32b). This incision continues also inside the nose.

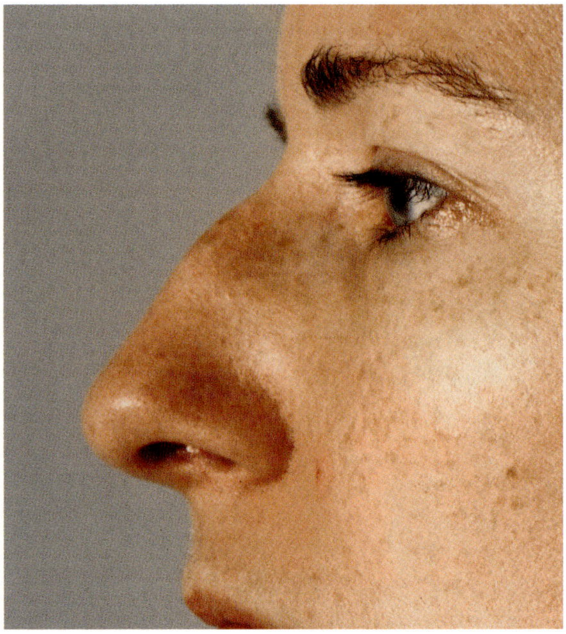

30a

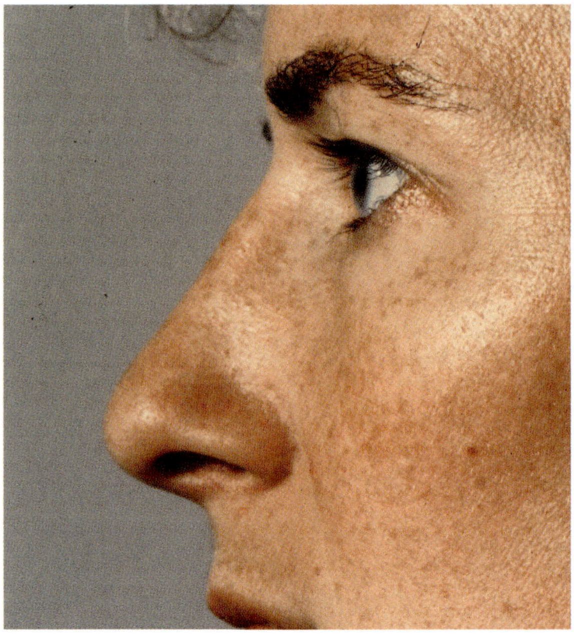

30b

30a,b Aesthetic rhinoplasty, before and after

The bony and the cartilaginous parts of the hump are removed (fig. 33). The nasal bones are brought together to form a narrowed nasal bridge (osteotomy; fig. 33). Cartilage is excised in the upper part of the nasal tip (cephalic part of the lateral crus of the alar cartilage) to reduce its size and to achieve a more harmonious contour (fig. 34).

To improve the angle between the upper lip and the base of the nose, a small amount of cartilage on the lower part of the septum is removed and thus the nasal tip is elevated (fig. 35).

If the nostrils are too widely flared at the base, they are brought closer together by removing a segment of the alar base (fig. 36 I / II). Following surgery, nasal pads are inserted in the nostrils. Tapes and an appropriate splint are applied to the nose to maintain the bone and the cartilage in the new shape (fig. 37).

When the nose must be built up, cartilage may be taken from other parts of the body – for instance from the ear or from a rib.

Aesthetic rhinoplasty requires between half an hour and one hour, depending upon the extent of surgery involved.

Postoperative considerations

Slight pain which may be experienced after surgery can be controlled easily by medication. Varying degrees of swelling and bruising around the eyes result within the first twenty-four hours after the operation, but will gradually decrease over a period of ten days.

The nasal packs are usually removed the second postoperative day and the nasal splint between ten and fourteen days after surgery. When the nasal splint is removed, the nose is still swollen and appears broad, particularly in the nasal tip area. Some subtle swelling of the nose will subside over a period of months. The final settling and softening may take six to twelve months, dur-

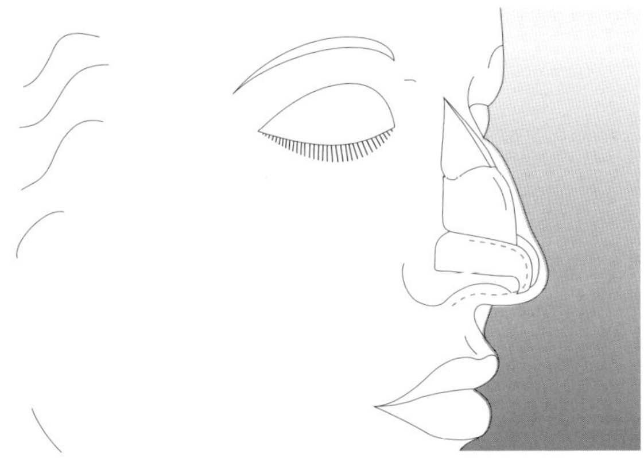

31

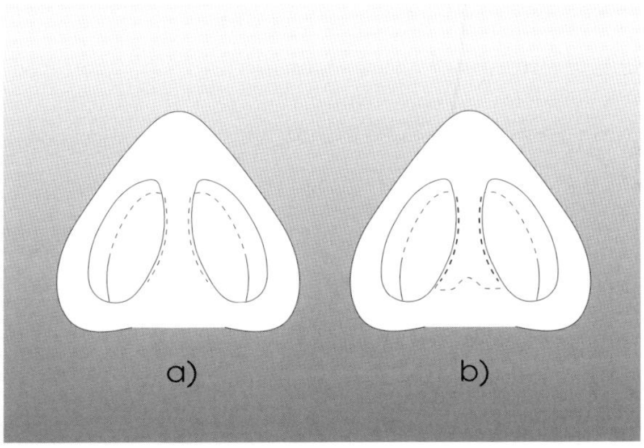

32a,b

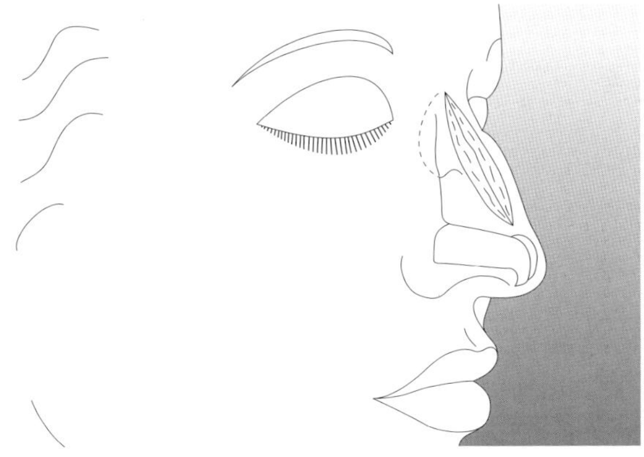

33

31 Incisions are usually made inside the nostrils

32a Incisions inside the nostrils

32b Rarely a small incision is made on the base of the nose (columella)

33 The nasal hump is removed; the bones are weakened at their base by osteotomy and brought together to form a narrower nasal bridge ing which time all final contour changes take place. The thicker the skin, the longer it takes for the nose to return to its definite shape. It usually takes several months until the final result can be fully appreciated. One should therefore not make any premature judgements. Patients may return to normal social activities within seven to fourteen days after surgery. Strenuous activities should be avoided for one to two weeks. Cosmetics may be used after removal of the splint. Great care must be taken that the nose is not injured in any way during a period of three weeks after the operation.

Important elements

An aesthetic rhinoplastiy can only be considered successful if the nose looks completely natural and perfectly harmonises with the other elements of the face so that surgery is not obvious.

Experience shows that the expected result is usually not obtained by one particular operative technique but only by the combination of various minor corrections. It is usually better to make small corrections than radical transformations which are rarely in harmony with the natural physiognomy of the patient.

Aesthetic rhinoplasty is carried out quite routinely during a face and neck lift. A minor rhinoplasty aimed at raising the tip of the nose of elderly patients helps to restore a youthful appearance of the face.

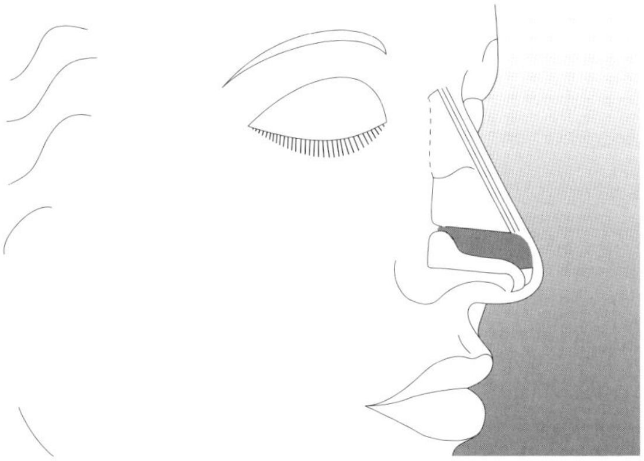

34

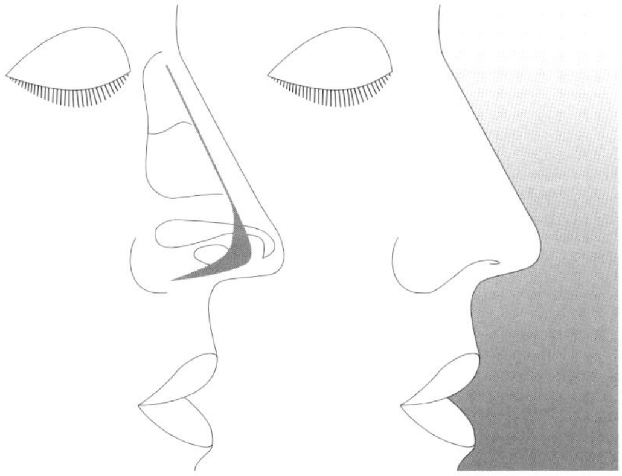

35

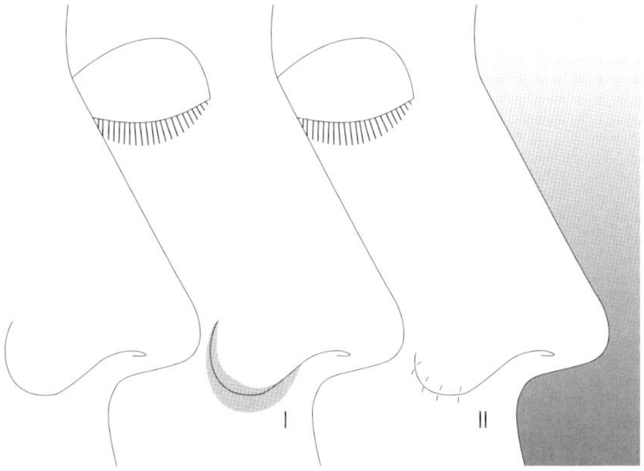

36

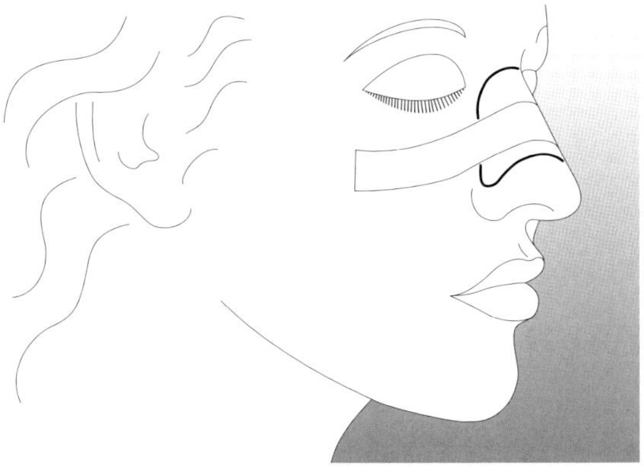

37

34 Cartilage is removed in the upper part of the nasal tip to reduce its size

35 To improve the angle between the base of the nose and the upper lip, a small amount of cartilage in the lower part of the septum is removed

36 To narrow the base of the nose, small skin wedges are removed (I). The scars are imperceptible (II)

37 Tape and nasal splint maintain bone and cartilage in the new shape

Facial Bone Structure Surgery

The beauty of the face is based on an ideal skeletal framework. The structural elements of the face - chin, cheekbones and forehead - have to be in harmony with each other to form what science and art call an "attractive countenance".

Facial bone structure surgery allows the contours of the face to be improved. It permits one to sculpt the bone structure of the face; either to add volume to certain regions or to reduce prominent parts of facial bone structures. The ultimate aim of these procedures is always to create a more harmonious relationship between the different elements of the face and to improve its overall appearance (fig. 38a,b).

Slightly prominent cheekbones constitute one of the essential components of facial beauty and harmony. Cheek augmentation procedures together with corrective procedures of the chin are the most frequently performed interventions on the facial bone structure. Surgical procedures aimed at changing the contour of the forehead, mostly in the region of the superciliary arch, or of the jaws are also possible, though rarely performed.

There are two surgical procedures for adding volume to the chin: insertion of an implant (mostly silicone) or forward advancement of the inferior part of the chin bone (sliding osteotomy). A slightly protuberant chin is reduced by burring the bone (figs. 38a,b, 41). A significant protuberance is usually corrected by sliding the inferior part of the chin backwards (sliding osteotomy). Very rarely cheek bones are too high in proportion to the rest of the face. In this case, cheek bone reduction is indicated.

Infection and haematomas are very uncommon and can be treated easily. If infection should occur with any implant, the device may have to be removed and replaced a few months later.

These procedures are usually performed under local anaesthesia with sedation, on an outpatient basis.

Chin Implants

An incision is made inside the lower lip or beneath the chin. The soft tissue is carefully detached from the bone in order to create space large enough for the appropriate implant. The chosen implant is anchored in the prepared

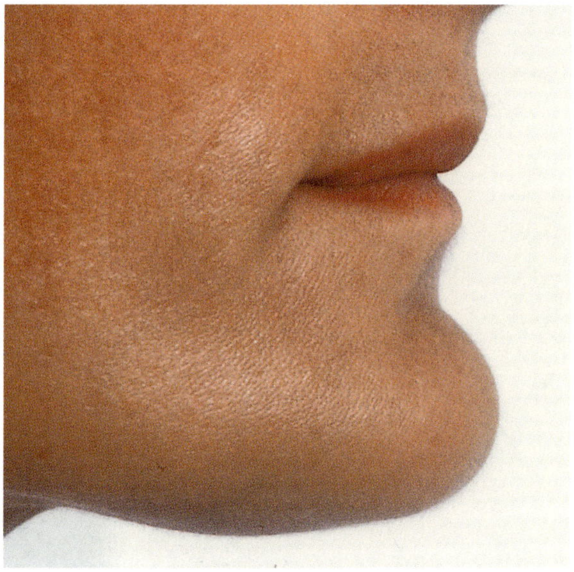

38a

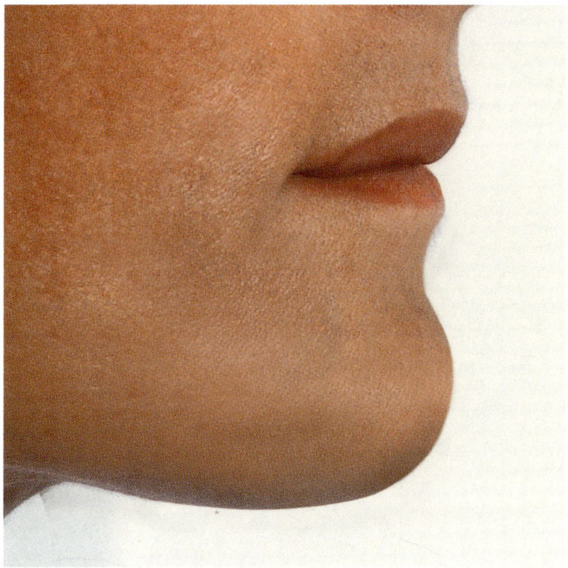

38b

38a,b Chin bone reduction by burring, before and after

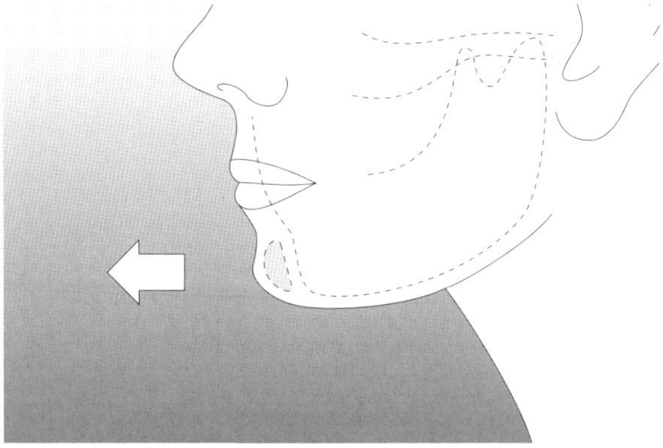

39

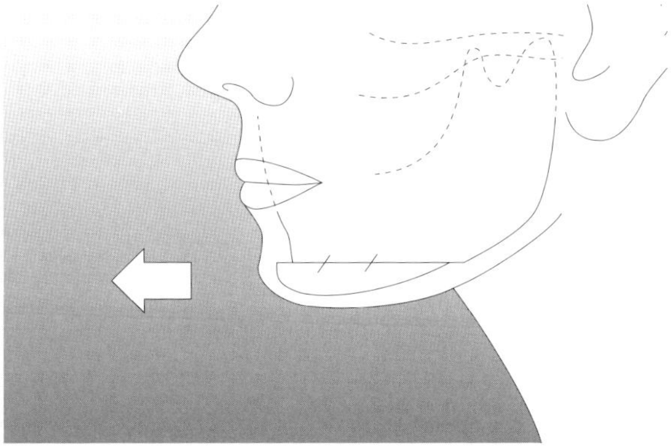

40

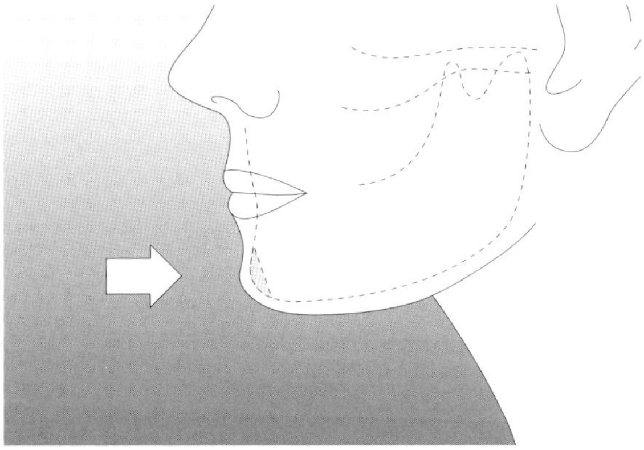

41

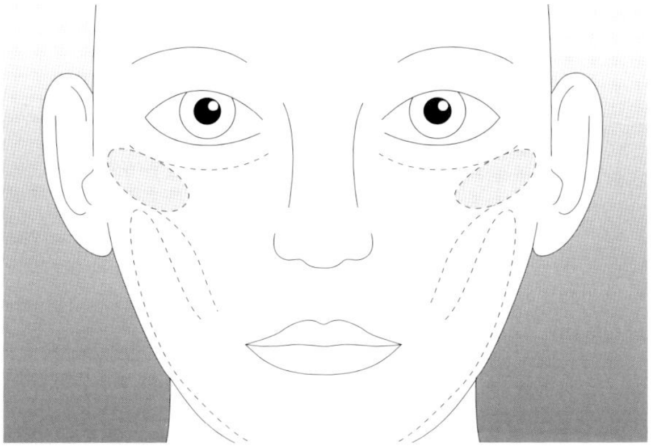

42

cavity with a synthetic dissolvable suture to maintain position and the wound is then closed (fig. 39).

Sliding Osteotomy of the Chin

In this technique, more rarely employed than the technique described before, the incision is usually placed inside the mouth (along the lower lip) to provide access to the chin bone. Using a sawing instrument, a horizontal cut is made through the bone. The lower portion of the separated bone is moved forward and wired in its new position before closing the wound (fig. 40).

Chin Reduction

An incision is made inside the mouth on the lower lip to provide access to the chin bone. The chin is reduced by burring of the bone with an electrically operated instrument (fig. 41).

For patients needing very substantial repositioning of the chin - which is extremely rare - a sliding osteotomy backwards (in the opposite direction from the procedure mentioned above) is performed.

Malar Implants

The incision is usually made inside the mouth between the upper gums and the cheek. The soft tissue is elevated, creating a pocket over the cheek bone and the adequate malar implant is inserted and possibly anchored with a synthetic dissolvable suture to maintain the implant in position and subsequently the wound is closed (fig. 42).

39 Augmentation of the chin by an implant

40 Advancement of the chin bone (sliding osteotomy)

41 Reduction of the chin bone by burring

42 Malar augmentation by implants

Reduction of Superciliary Arches and Lower Jaw Implants

These types of operation are not very common. The edges of the superciliary arch can be reduced by burring of the bone protuberance. Jaw implants are placed directly on the jawbone to create a stronger, more defined jawline.

These different surgical procedures last between half an hour and one hour depending upon the extent of surgery.

Postoperative considerations

Swelling, bruises and some numbness in the operated regions are very common and begin to subside three to four days after surgery and disappear gradually during the following weeks.

Most patients can resume their usual activities within two or three days and their social life within seven to ten days. Strenuous exercises should be avoided for two weeks.

Important elements

Augmentation procedures of the chin and cheek bone with implants not only provide a more harmonious balance to the face but often contribute also to its youthfulness.

An understanding of the unique balance of the different components of facial architecture is the key to a correct evaluation and diagnosis of facial disharmony. The different elements of the face should always be viewed together and not in isolation. Drastic changes are usually not a reasonable objective because they are rarely compatible with the whole contour of the face.

Aesthetic Otoplasty

Aesthetic surgery can improve the shape or size of the ears if they are in disproportion with other facial features or can improve the positioning, if they protrude more than normal. Sometimes in an attempt to improve the harmony of the whole ear it is indicated to change the size and shape of the earlobe.

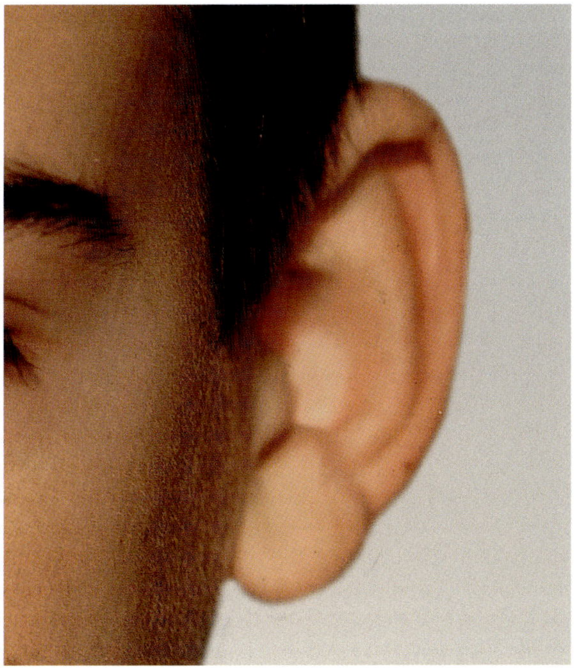

43a

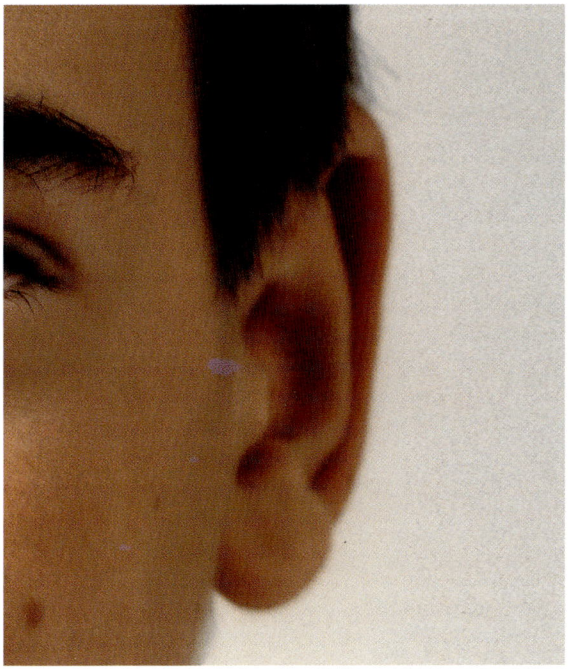

43b

43a,b Correction of protruding ears or aesthetic otoplasty, before and after

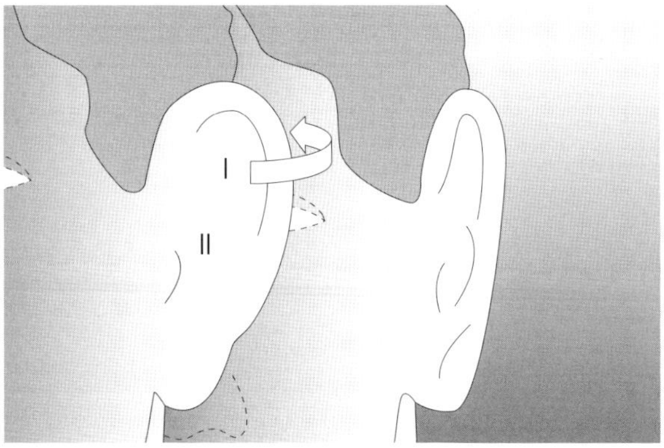

44

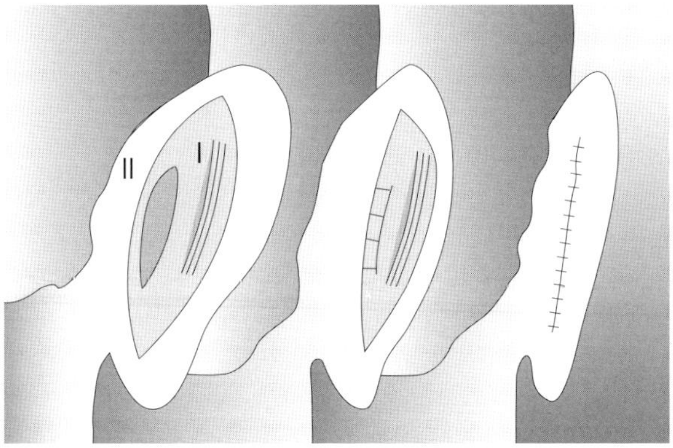

45

The most common aesthetic procedure on the ears is aesthetic otoplasty or the correction of protruding ears (fig. 43a,b).

There may be two different reasons why ears protrude: either the shell-shaped curve of the ear (concha or outer ear; fig. 44/II) is too large, or the cartilaginous fold (antihelix; fig. 44/I) inside the outer edge of the ear is under-developed or non-existent. These two conditions are often combined. The operating technique is therefore determined by the type of deformity. Otoplasty can sometimes be simple and at other times be quite complex. The aim is to always obtain a natural shape of the ear and a natural position without being set too far back. Surgery is possible as early as the age of four or five and at any age for adults.

The scars behind the ear are concealed in the skin folds. In exceptional cases a scar may grow thicker and wider owing to a significant scarring reaction (hypertrophic scar). In some very rare cases the corrected ears may reveal a small deformation of the cartilage that has been operated on, or they may protrude again slightly. In this case, a slight correction can be carried out a few weeks or months later.

In general an aesthetic otoplasty to correct protruding ears is performed under local anaesthesia with sedation on an outpatient basis.

Surgical procedure

The method employed depends on the cause of the protrusion (fig. 44). Usually a combination of two techniques is necessary to obtain an optimal result. As a rule, if the fold on the outer edge of the ear is not properly formed or non-existent, one of the techniques is to make an incision at the back of the ear and fold the cartilage to reshape the ear (fig. 45/I). Sometimes the same effect can be achieved by scraping the cartilage in front of the ear through a tiny incision in order to weaken it and then folding it back with special internal stitches. If the shape and form of the concha is the cause of the protrusion or contributes together with the missing antihelix fold to the protrusion, a wedge of cartilage is removed from behind the ear and the cartilage is sutured (figs. 44/II, 45/II).

An aesthetic otoplasty requires between three quarters of an hour and one hour, depending upon the extent of surgery involved.

Postoperative considerations

Depending on the type of operation, a light head bandage must be worn during sleep for two to three weeks. Swelling and bruises will gradually disappear within a few weeks. Most adults will be able to go back to work within two

44 Aesthetic Otoplasty. Remodelling of a cartilaginous fold (antihelix) (I) and removal of cartilage from the concha (II)
45 Aesthetic Otoplasty. In general, an incision is made behind the ear. The cartilage is incised and folded back in the outer part of the ear (antihelix) (I), a wedge of cartilage is removed from the concha (II). Usually both procedures are combined The scar is usually thin and invisible, situated in the skin fold behind the ear

social activities. The postoperative oedema is also quite significant after a vermillion advancement or lip reduction. The sutures can be removed four to five days after the intervention. Adequate make-up may be applied since the scar remains red for several months. The patient can usually resume a normal social life one week to ten days after surgery.

Important Elements

Lip enlargement has been fashionable for a few decades. From Marilyn Monroe to Sophia Loren and Greta Garbo, sensual lips have been a key element of seductiveness and beauty. Lip enlargement can often enhance the youthful appearance of the face. However, the shape and volume of the lips should always be in harmony with the other elements of the face.

Even though a lip augmentation by injectable products and micro lipofilling is a relatively simple medical treatment, experience, skill and artistic sense are required in order to achieve an optimal result. Vermillion advancement and lip reduction can only lead to perfect results if such an intervention has been precisely planned after a careful aesthetic assessment and by studying the static and dynamic anatomy of the patients' face. The amount of tissue excision has to be determined with extreme accuracy.

Non biodegradable filling substances should never be used for lip augmentation because they can give rise to chronic inflammatory tissue reactions and even hardening, sometimes occurring many years after the injection was performed.

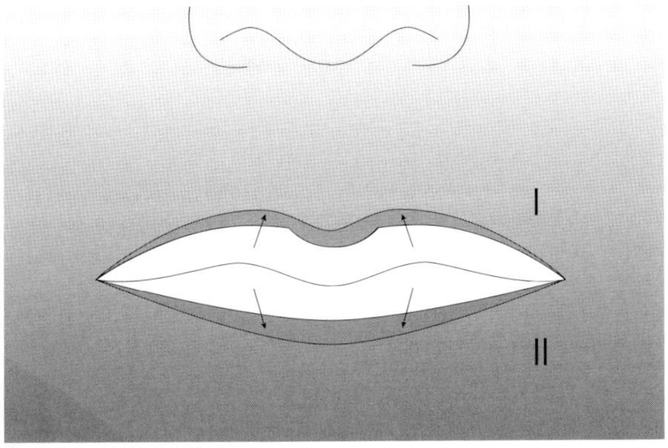

48

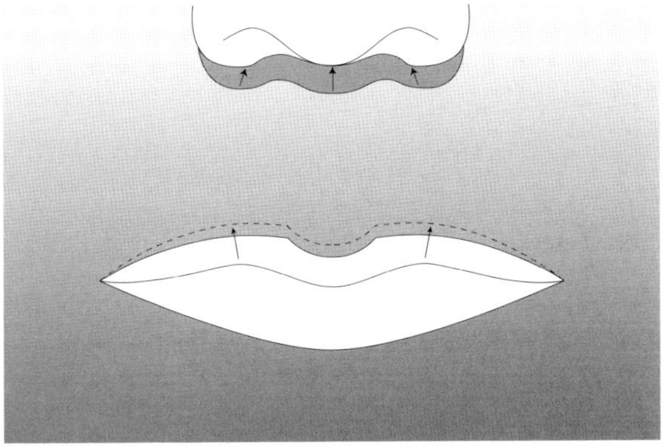

49

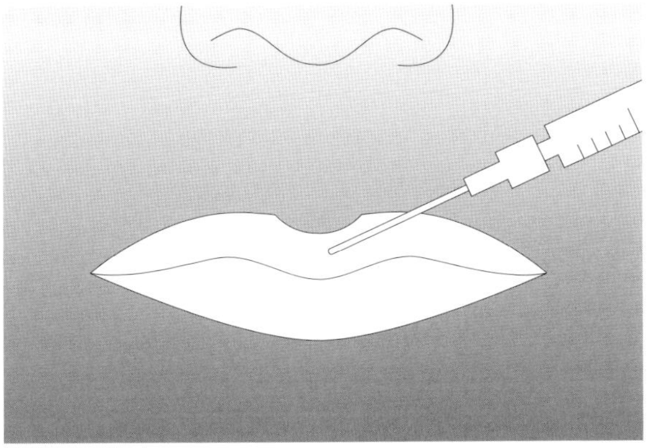

50

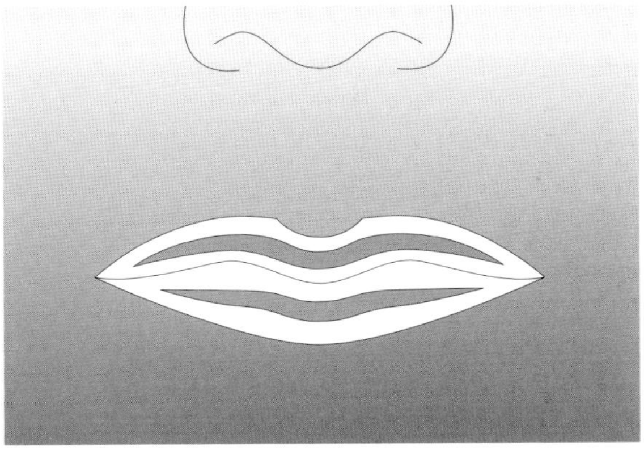

51

48 I/II Vermillion advancement of the upper and lower lip by excision of a skin wedge at the outside of the vermillion

49 Upper lip lift by skin excision on the base of the nose

50 Lip augmentation by injectable products or micro lipofilling

51 Lip augmentation by dermal grafts

Pre- and Postoperative Considerations

Good physical health is a significant advantage to ensure the best possible result. Therefore it is best to plan the operation when one is in optimal physical condition. Firmly established emotional stability is also important before any aesthetic surgery is undertaken. Overall equilibrium will greatly help to ensure success. By following rigorously the instructions given, it is possible to influence the entire course of the healing process in a positive way.

Patients should try to achieve their ideal weight if they are overweight. A weight reduction will improve the harmony of the whole body to a marked degree.

It is also advisable to stop smoking at least three weeks before surgery. This minimizes the risk of bleeding and of delayed and improper wound healing. Nicotine has a constrictive effect on the blood vessels which reduces tissue oxygenation. This can impede the scarring process and may even cause necrosis of skin tissue in operations involving significant detachment of skin.

Certain pain-killing drugs, particularly aspirin-containing medications and alcoholic beverages, should not be taken for at least three weeks prior to surgery. Aspirin and alcohol can cause significant intra-operative bleeding. Aspirin interferes with normal blood coagulation and alcohol causes a significant vasodilation effect.

Caution is also required when using other substances, such as vitamin E in high doses, certain natural substances such as Ginseng, Gingko biloba, spices and other designated medications.

These recommendations are also valid for the first few days after the intervention. All this is as important to achieving the best result as is the excellent performance of the surgeon.

The length of convalescence depends on the type and scale of the operation (see post-operative schedule).

After aesthetic procedures, such as a forehead, face- and neck lift or a blepharoplasty, which cause significant swelling, it is advisable to sleep with the head slightly raised, and to apply ice packs to the swollen parts of the face for the first few days. Lymphatic drainage and daily physical exercise, especially walking, considerably facilitate the reabsorption of the post-operative oedema.

Patients may resume normal social activities seven to ten days after a forehead lift, ten to fourteen days after a face- and neck lift, seven to ten days after a mini lift or a minimal incision face lift, five to seven days after blepharoplasty and five to ten days after surface treatments (see post-operative schedule, figs. 52–62).

As patients generally wish to resume their usual activities as soon as possible, the use of specific camouflage cosmetics is suggested in order to mask the undesirable postoperative effects. There are three types of hypoallergenic masking products: concealers to mask red scars, green colour correctors to cover yellow or reddish skin discolorations, and contouring products to disguise the swelling of certain parts of the face (figs. 52–66).

Normal make-up should not be used before all the staples and sutures have been removed and the wounds have completely closed again.

As a rule, make-up can be used one week after rejuvenative facial surgery and one to two weeks after a surface treatment, which is the time it takes for the scabs to disappear completely, see post-operative schedule.

Post-operative schedule

Type of intervention	Duration (hours)	Camouflage cosmetics/make-up after (day)	Ordinary physical activity without strain (walking, etc.) after (day)	Normal physical activity after (day)	Resumption of social life after (day)
Upper blepharoplasty	½–¾	4th–5th	2nd	3rd	5th–7th
Lower blepharoplasty	½–¾	3rd–4th	2nd	3rd	5th–7th
Forehead and brow lift	1–1¼	3rd–4th	3rd	5th	7th–10th
Neck and face lift	2–2½	5th–7th	3rd	5th–8th	10th–14th
Minimal incision face lift	1½–2hr	3rd–5th	3rd	4th–6th	7th–10th
Micro liposuction/liposculpture	¼–½	3rd–5th	2nd	3rd	5th–8th
Surface treatments (dermabrasion, peeling, laser) according to technique, surface and depth	¼–1hr	3rd–10th	1st	3rd	5th–10th
Botulinum toxin (Vistabel®, Botox®)	max. ¼	0	0	0	
Injectable products (collagen, hyaluronic acid)	max. ¼	0	0	0	0
Micro lipofilling	¼–¾	1st	1st	3rd–5th	3rd–7th
Rhinoplasty (according to type)	½–1hr	5th–10th	1st	7th–10th	7th–14th
Chin augmentation/enlargement a) Implant b) Osteotomy	 ¼–½ ¾–1hr	 2nd–3rd 4th–6th	 2nd 3rd	 5th–7th 5th–7th	 5th–8th 7th–10th
Chin reduction	½	3rd–4th	2nd	5th–7th	7th–10th
Cheek augmentation by implants	½–¾	2nd–3rd	2nd	5th–7th	7th–10th
Aesthetic otoplasty	¾–1hr	5th–7th	2nd	3rd–5th	2nd–10th
Lip lift	½–¾	5th–7th	2nd	4th–5th	7th–10th
Lip reduction	½–¾	3rd–4th	2nd	4th–5th	7th–10th
Lip augmentation by injectable products	max. ¼	0	0	0	0
Lip augmentation by micro lipofilling or dermal graft	¼–½	2nd	1st	3rd–5th	5th–7th

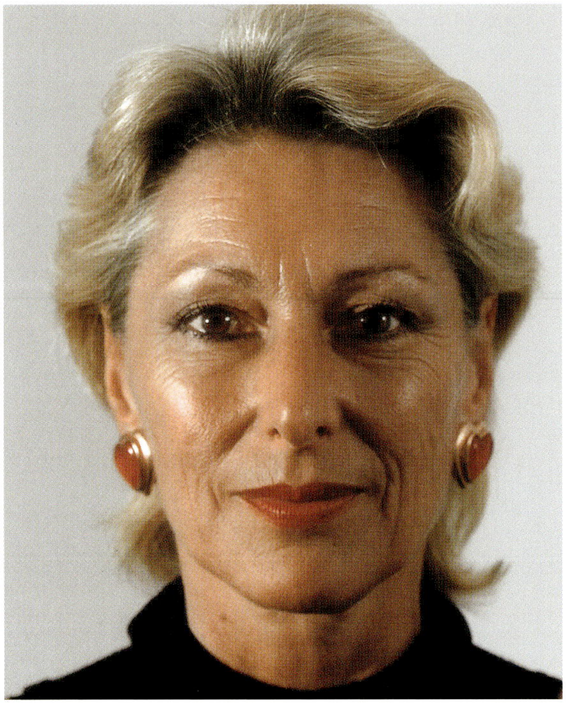

52a

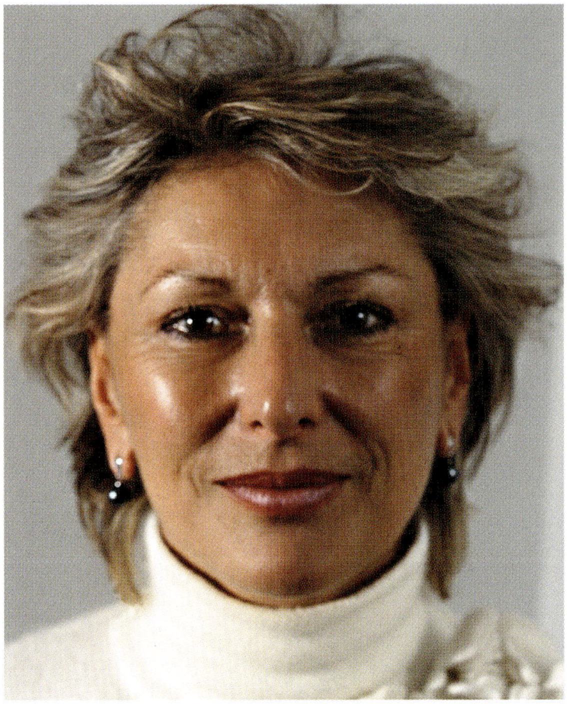

53a

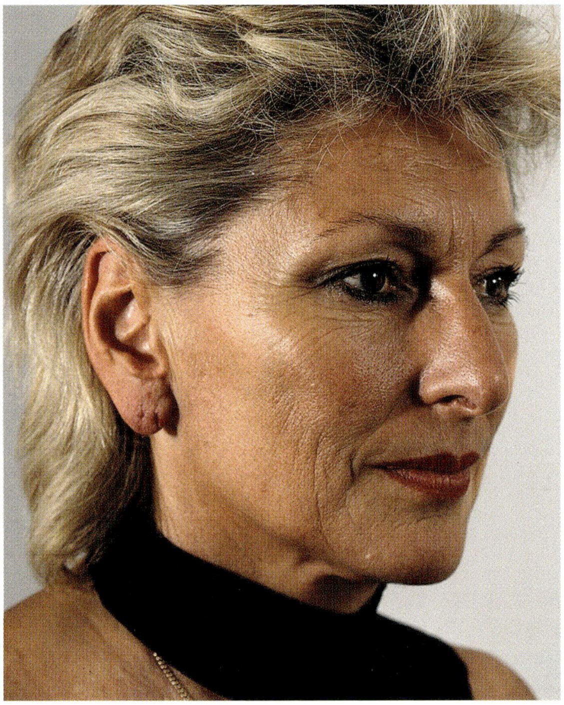

52b

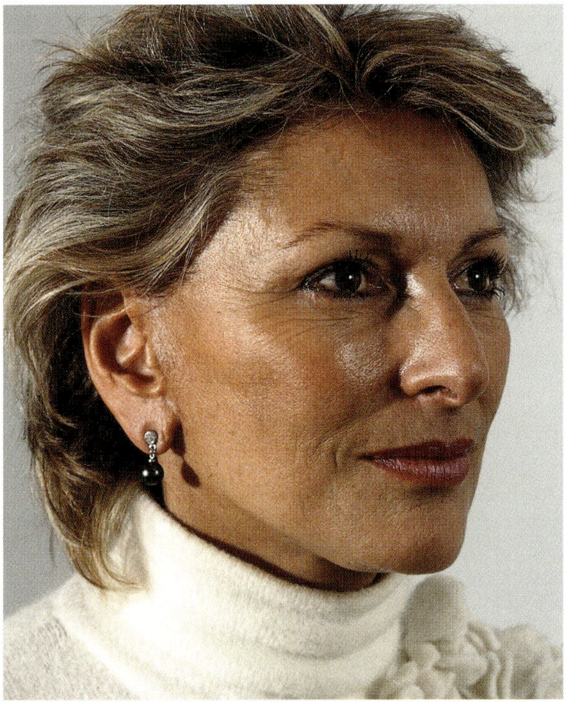

53b

52a,b Before surgery

53a,b 4 months after temporal lift, neck- and face lift with SMAS and platysma plasty, upper and lower blepharoplasty, micro lipofilling of upper and lower lip, Vistabel® (botulinum toxin) in fronto-orbital region

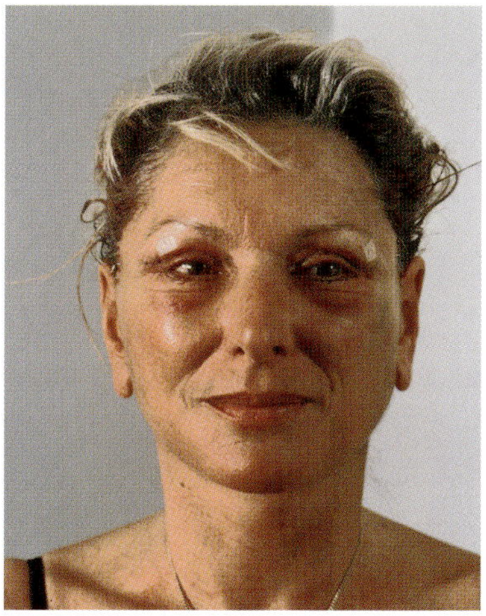
54a

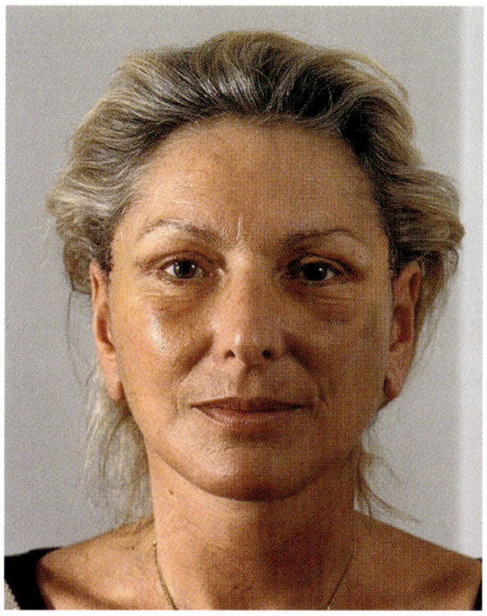
55a

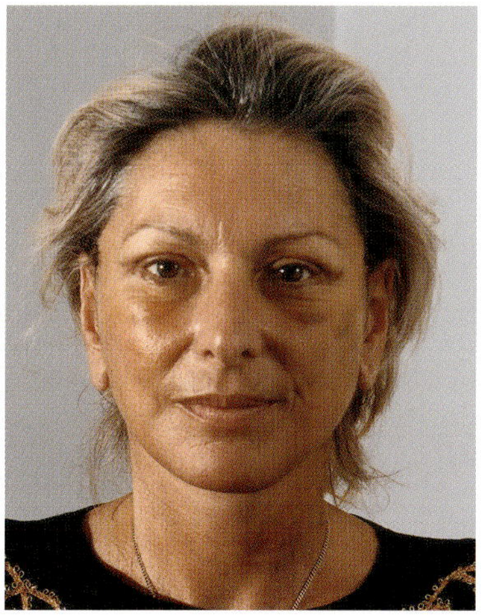
56a

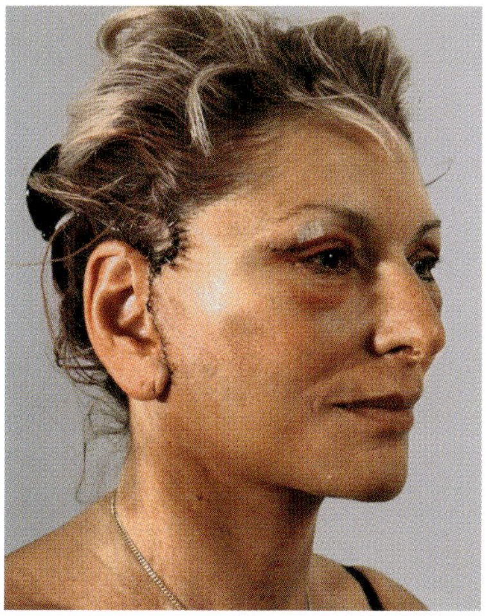
54b

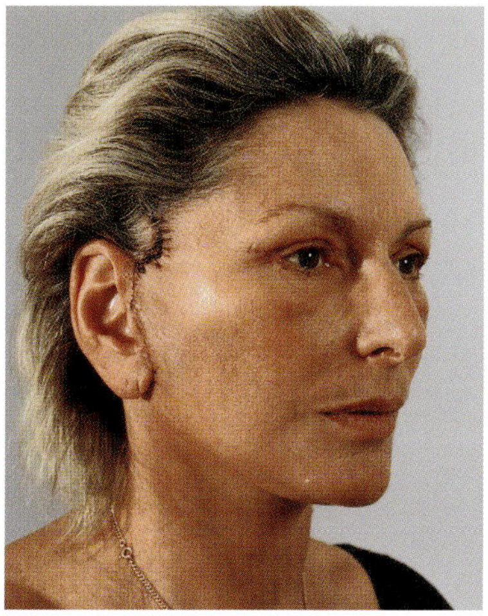
55b

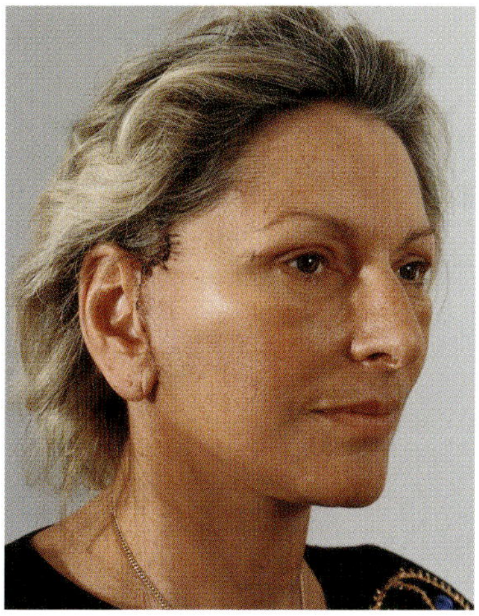
56b

54a,b 1st post-operative day, without masking products, without make-up
55a,b 3rd post-operative day, without masking products, without make-up
56a,b 5th post-operative day, without masking products, without make-up

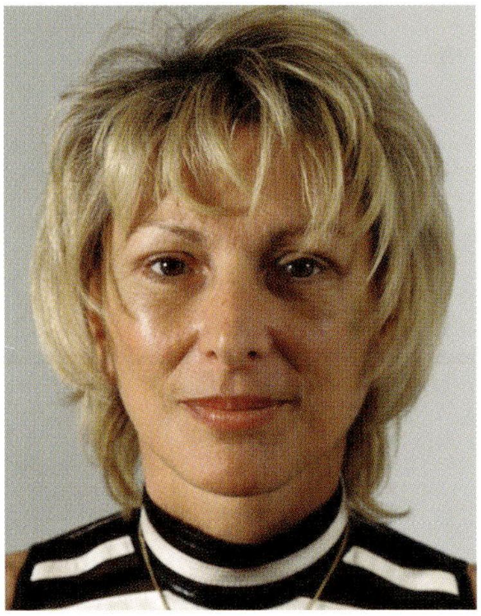

57a

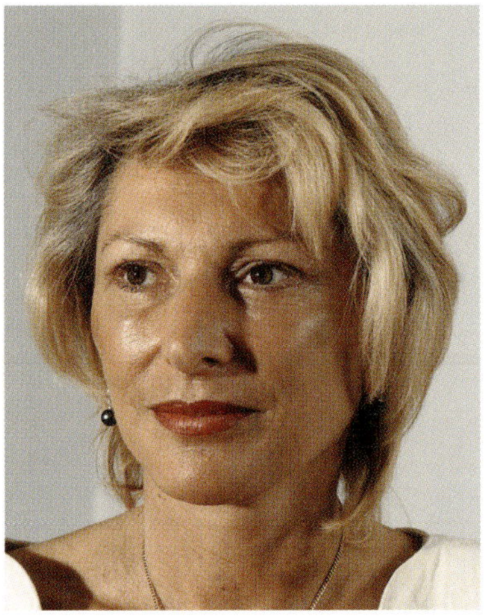

58a

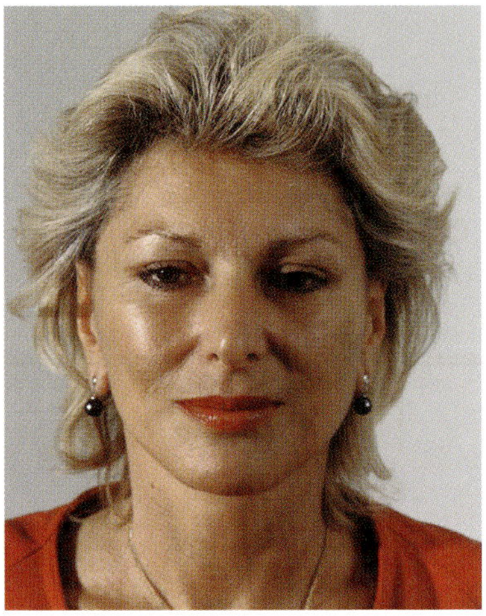

59a

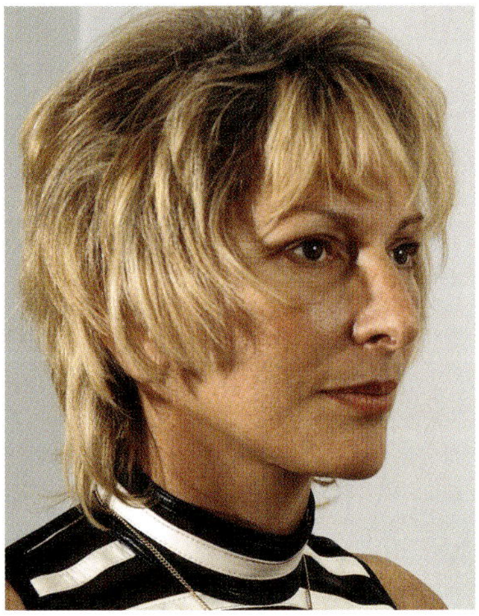

57b

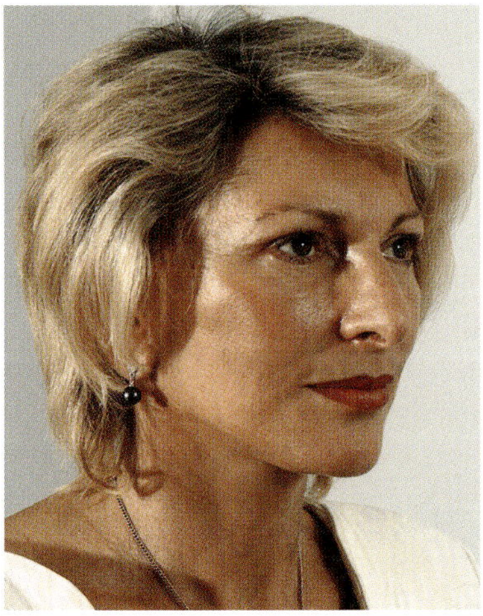

58b

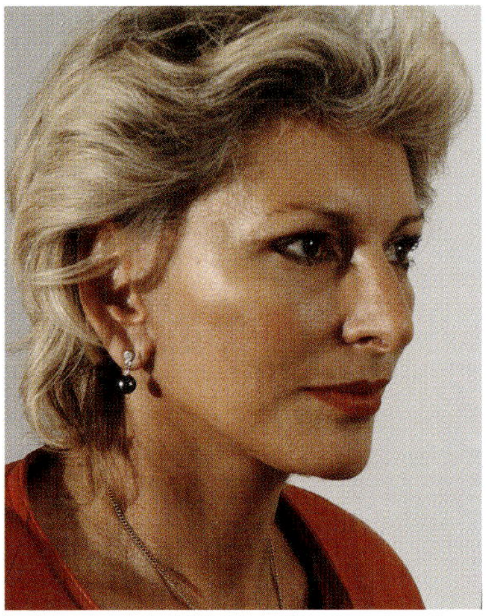

59b

57a,b 7th post-operative day, with masking products and make-up

58a,b 10th post-operative day, with masking products and make-up

59a,b 4th post-operative day, without masking products, with make-up

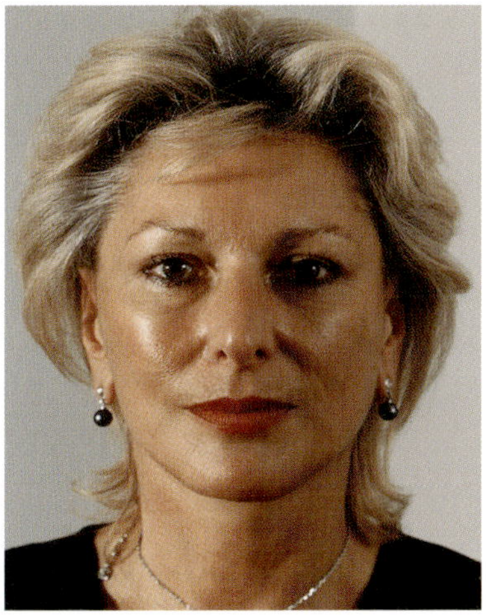

60a

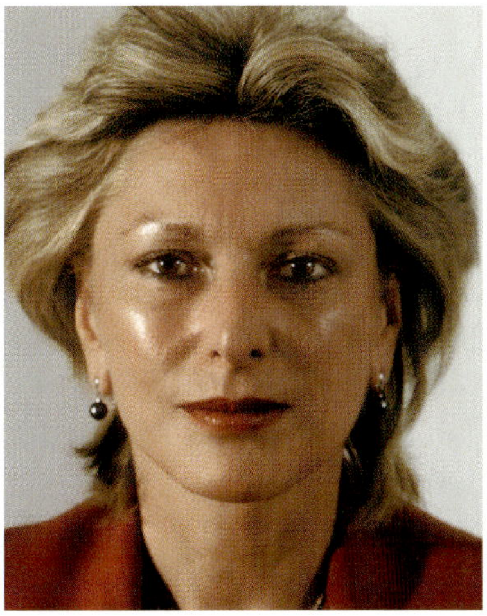

61a

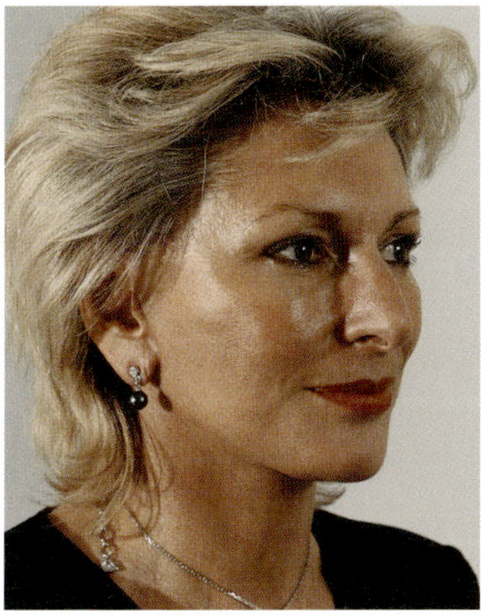

60b

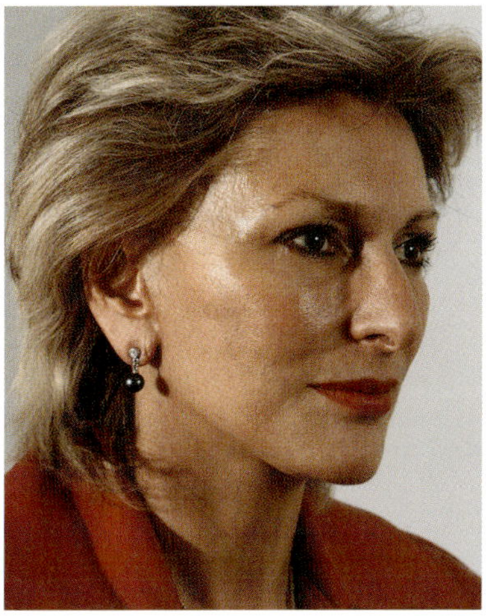

61b

60a,b 1 month after the operation
61a,b 2 months after the operation

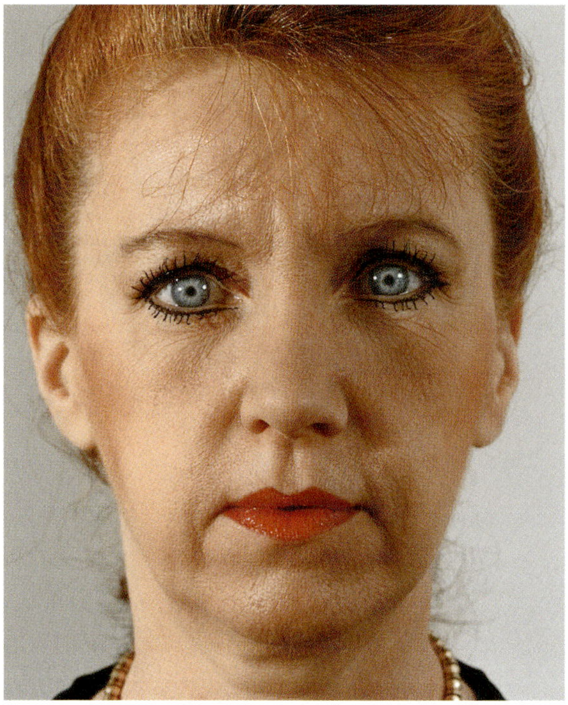
62a

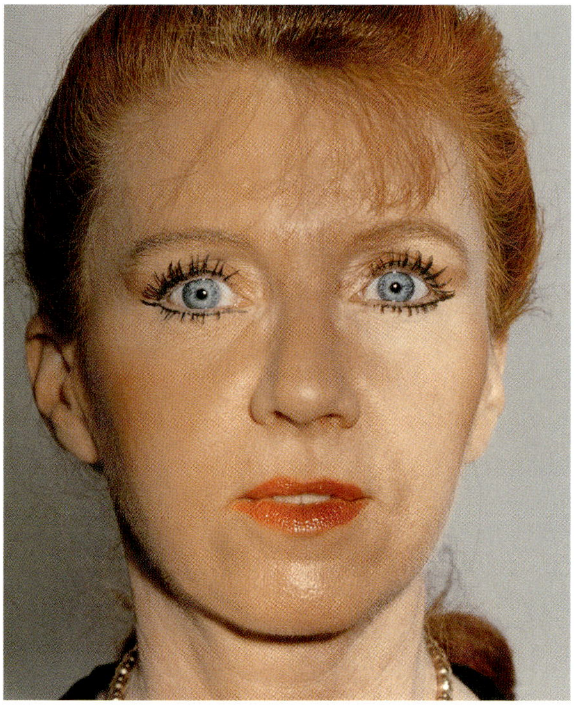
63a

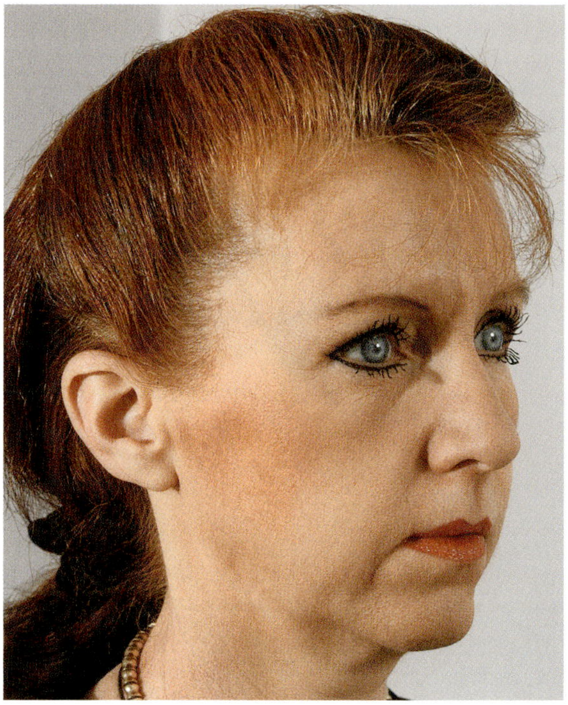
62b

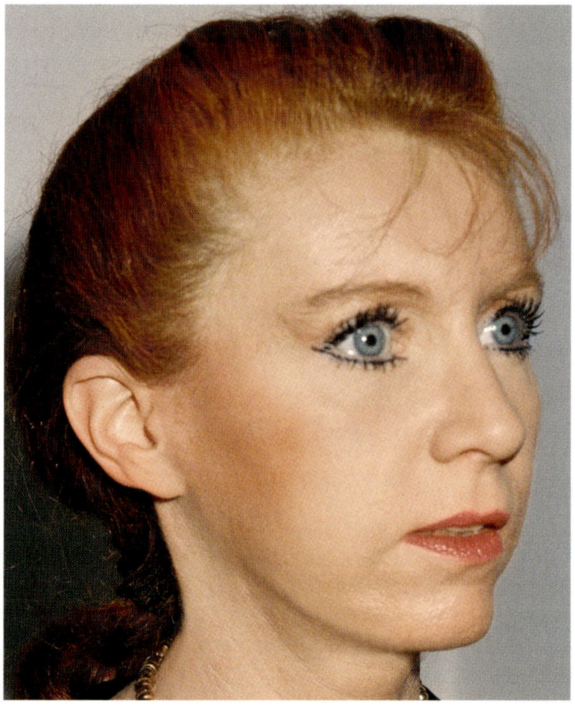
63b

62a,b Before surgery
63a,b 4 months after temporal lift, neck- and face lift with SMAS and platysma plasty, upper and lower blepharoplasty

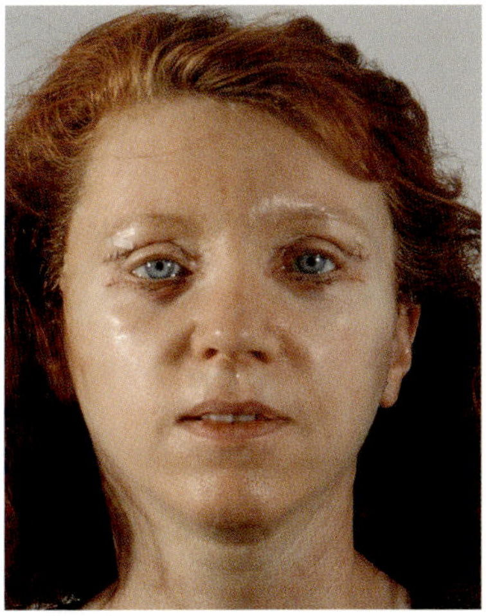

64a

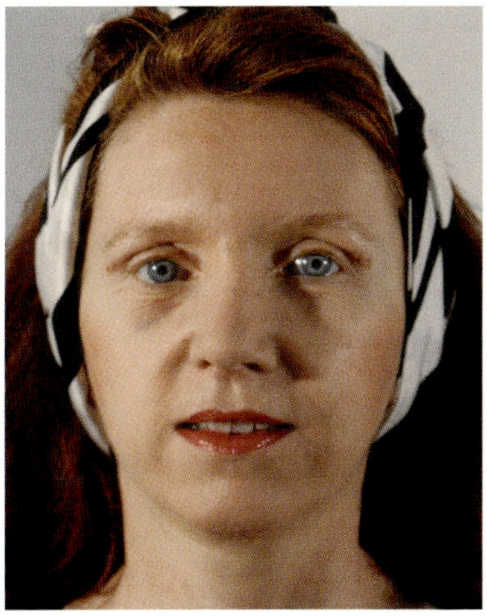

65a

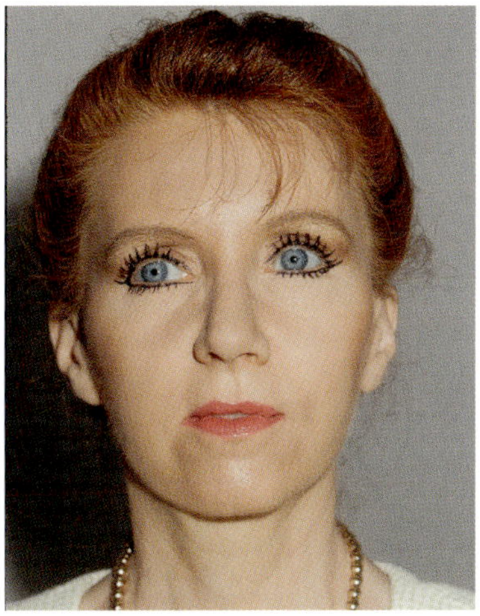

66a

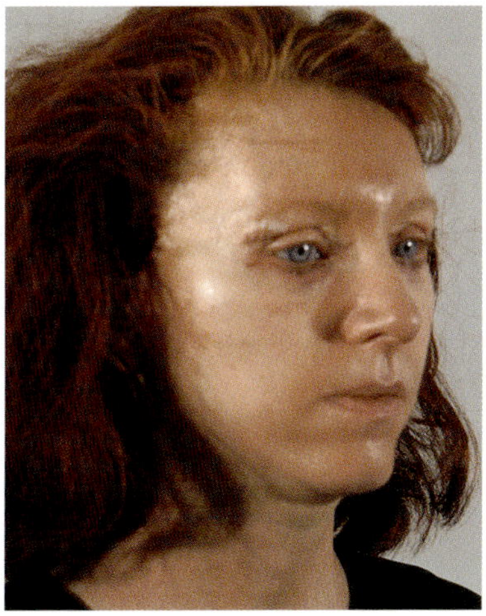

64b

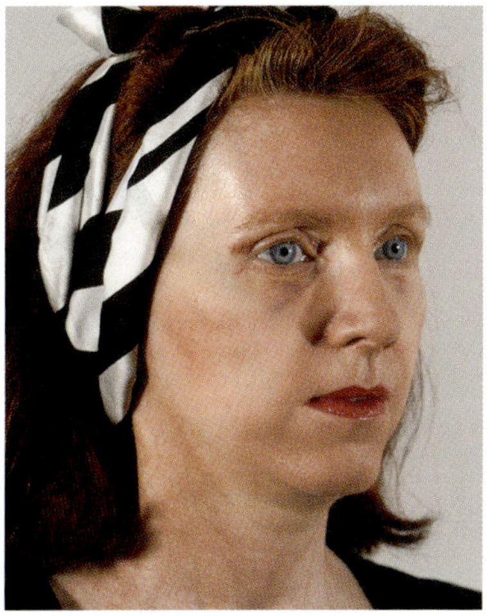

65b

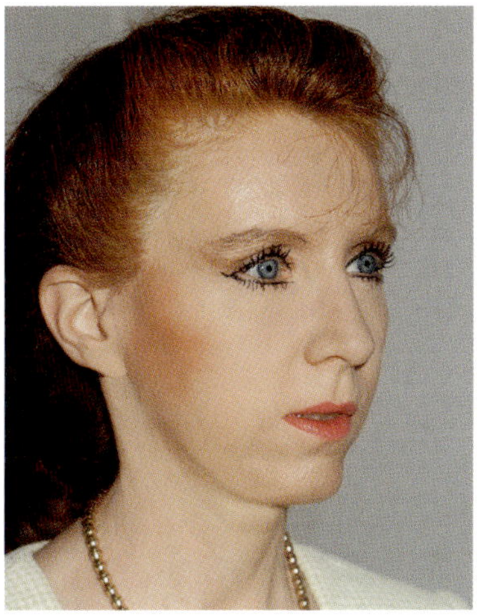

66b

64a,b 2nd post-operative day without masking products, without make-up
65a,b 7th post-operative day, with masking products and make-up
66a,b 14th post-operative day, without masking products, with make-up

The Quest for Perfection in Facial Rejuvenation

Optimal treatment for the surgical rejuvenation of the face is based on an appropriate choice from a wide range of surgical procedures and aesthetic treatments, each of them modified according to the patient's individual need. The surgeon must take into account the particular features of each face in order to achieve the most natural, harmonious and long-lasting result. Facial rejuvenation requires an equal reversal of all components contributing to ageing in order to guarantee a harmonious and natural result. Accurate pre-operative planning based on a precise diagnosis of the static and dynamic anatomy of the patient, along with a profound knowledge of facial aesthetics, is of fundamental importance.

Every successful result of aesthetic facial rejuvenation surgery is based primarily on the harmonization of the overall facial physiognomy. An aesthetic intervention in the frontal and orbital region must therefore usually be combined with corresponding operating procedures in the central and lower parts of the face and in the neck region – and vice versa. For the intervention described hereafter, the minor temporal lift (which raises slightly the temporal region and the outer part of the eyebrows), was combined with a face lift and repositioning of the deep tissue layers (SMAS), a partial neck lift with tightening of the platysma muscle, a minor correction of the lower eyelid and a superficial facial peeling of the upper and lower lip (figs. 1a,b).

The aesthetic surgeon has to take into account a host of tiny details in every facial rejuvenation procedure. I will describe a few of them taking the example of the patient shown first (figs. 1a,b): The eyebrows have to be positioned so as to enhance the overall harmony of the physiognomy. In this patient only the outer part of the eyebrow and orbital region was raised slightly (figs. 1a,b), no upper blepharoplasty was indicated. The natural hairline in the temple region and occipital region should not be moved by the operation so that there is no limitation for hair styles (figs. 1a,b).

To prevent any unnatural tension in the face and neck regions, the direction of skin repositioning has to be determined carefully. In order to achieve the most harmonious and most durable contour change in the cheek and neck region and an optimal correction of the nasolabial folds and the folds in the anterior-cheek region on this patient, I performed a SMAS flap with a posterior-superior rotation in the face region and a platysma suspension in the neck region (figs. 1a,b; see also Chapter on face- and neck lifts, pp. 81–85). The ear lobe is located in the extension of the longitudinal axis of the ear, as before surgery (figs. 1a,b). It should never be pulled forwards, backwards or downwards. The structures of the ear, in particular the cartilage in front of the ear, the tragus, should not show the slightest deviation from the anatomical conditions prior to the intervention (figs. 1a,b). The incisions should be positioned in such a way that the scars are completely invisible (figs. 1a,b). The distance between the edges of the upper and lower eyelids must be exactly the same as before surgery (fig. 1a), etc.

Only a perfect combination of a variety of different, safe and effective rejuvenative procedures, adapted specifically to the individual biological and anatomical conditions of each patient, will yield an optimal, natural and long-lasting result (see surgical sketches with pre-and postoperative photographs, figs. 2–33).

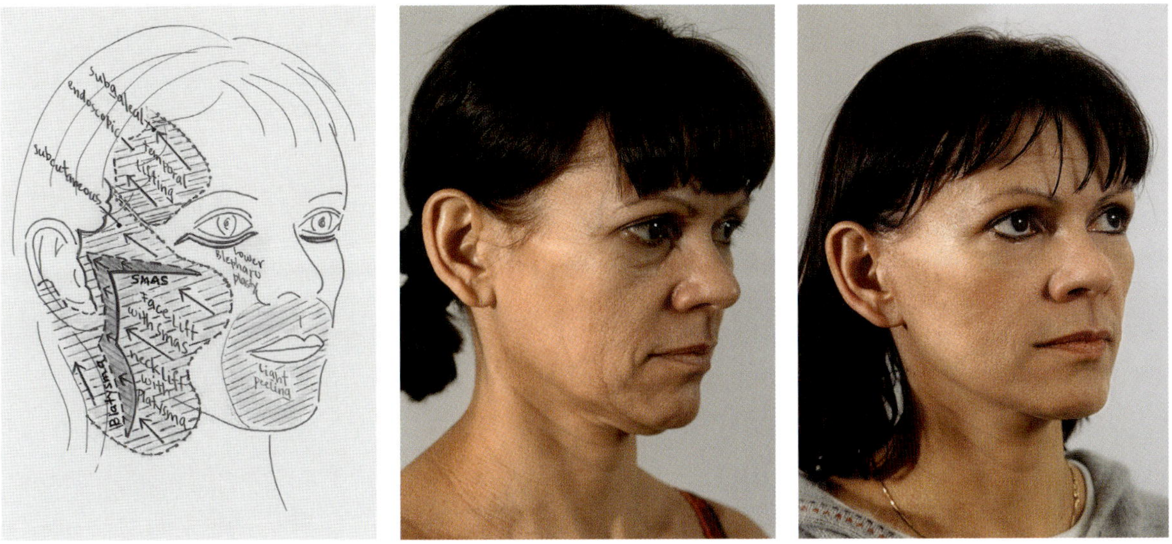

1a Preparatory surgical sketches (semi-profile). Before and after. Temporal lift, lower blepharoplasty, face and neck lift with SMAS and platysmaplasty, light peeling of the upper and lower lips

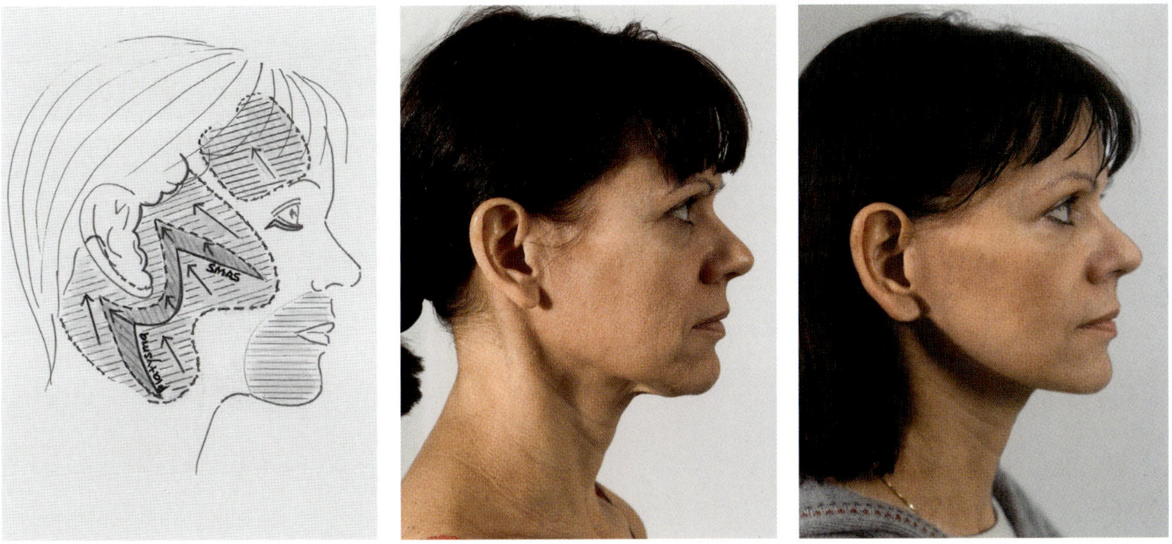

1b Preparatory surgical sketches (profile). Before and after. Endoscopic temple lift, lower blepharoplasty, face and neck lift with SMAS and platysmaplasty, light peeling of the upper and lower lips

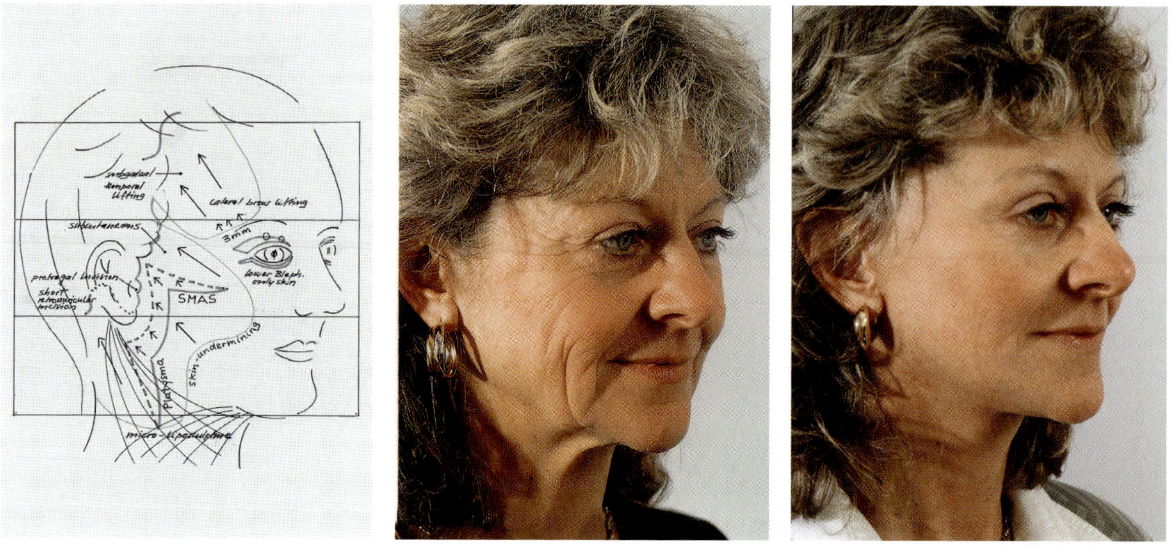

2 Temple lift, face and neck lift with SMAS, platysmaplasty and micro liposculpture, upper and lower blepharoplasty

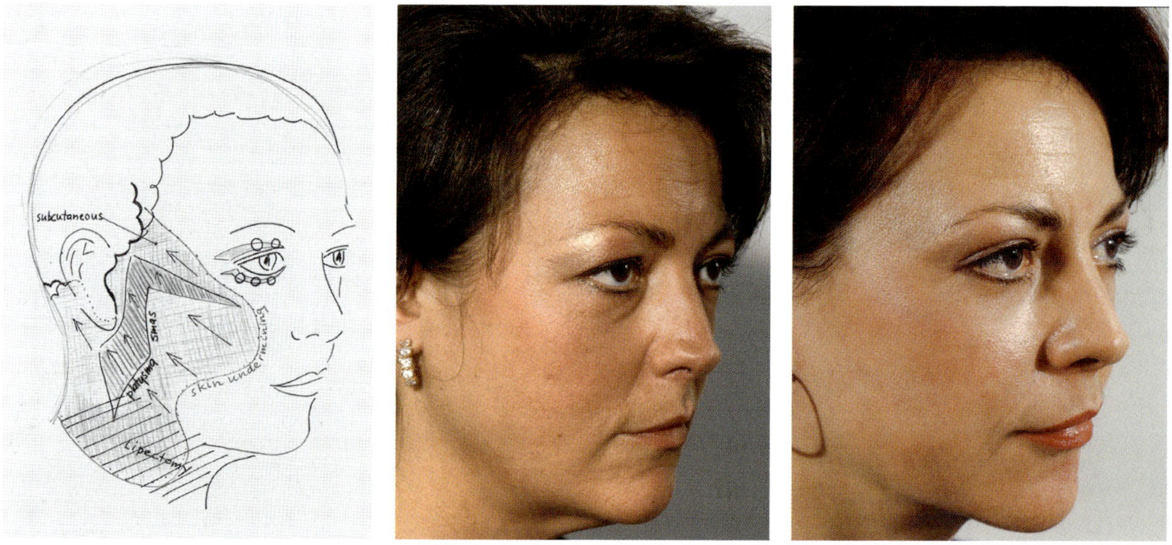

3 Face and neck lift with SMAS and platysmaplasty, upper and lower blepharoplasty

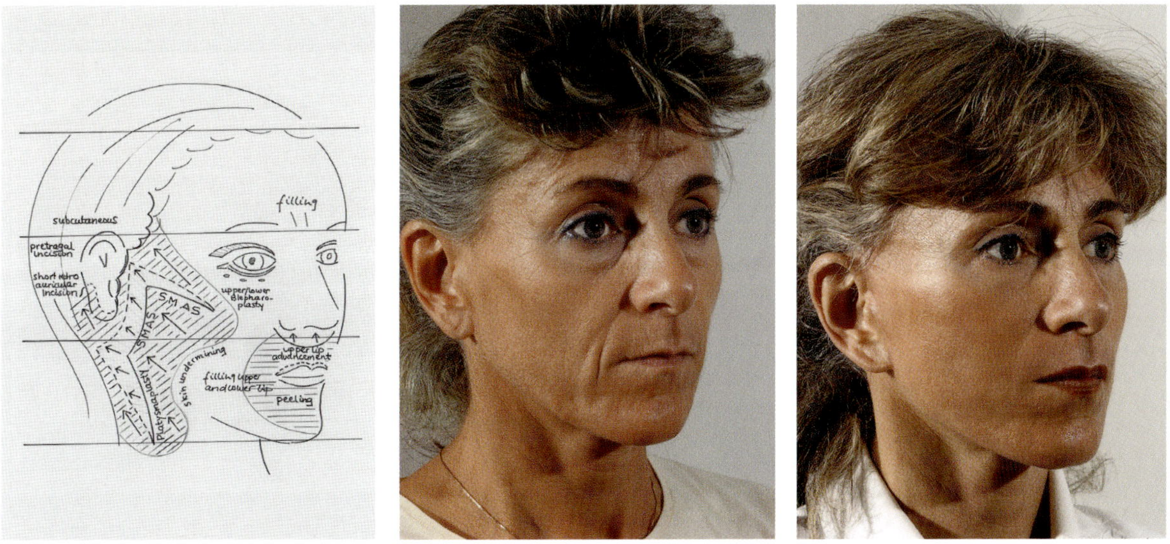

4 Face and neck lift with SMAS and platysmaplasty, upper and lower blepharoplasty, upper lip lift, filling of frown lines and the upper and lower lips, peeling of upper and lower lips

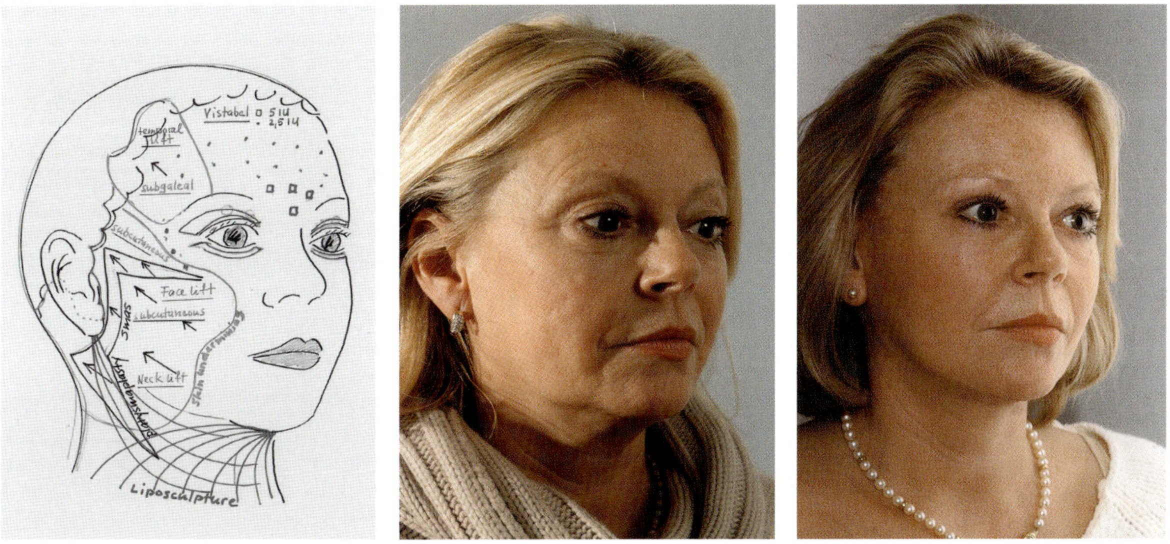

5 Temple lift, face lift with SMAS, neck lift with platysmaplasty and micro liposculpture, upper and lower blepharoplasty, injections of Vistabel® (botulinum toxin) in frontal region and outer orbital region

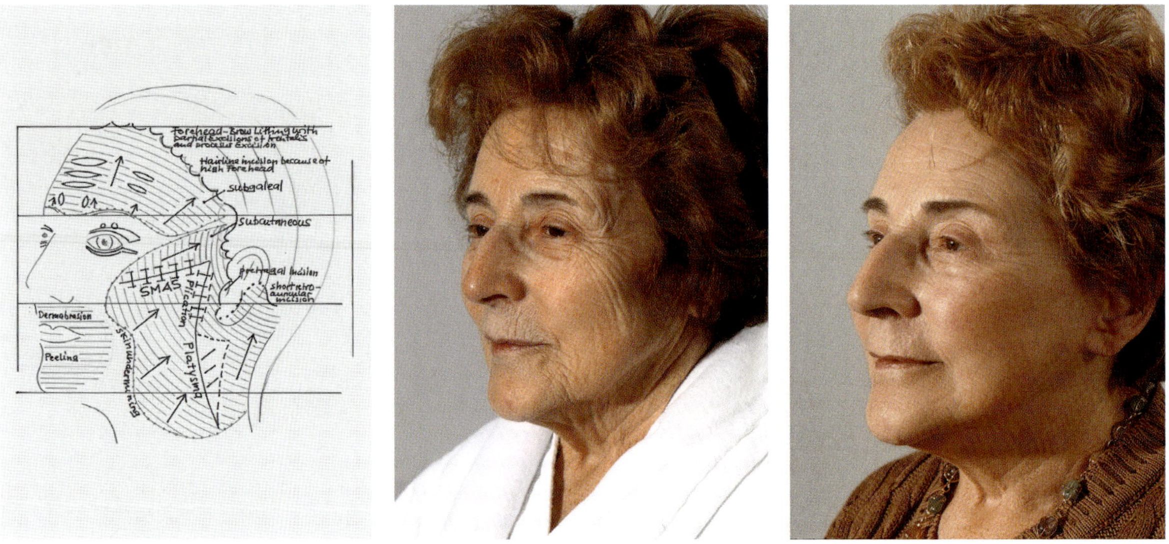

6 Forehead and eyebrow lift with myoplasties, face lift with SMAS-plication, neck lift with platysmaplasty and micro liposculpture, upper and lower blepharoplasty, dermabrasion of upper and lower lips, peeling of lower lip

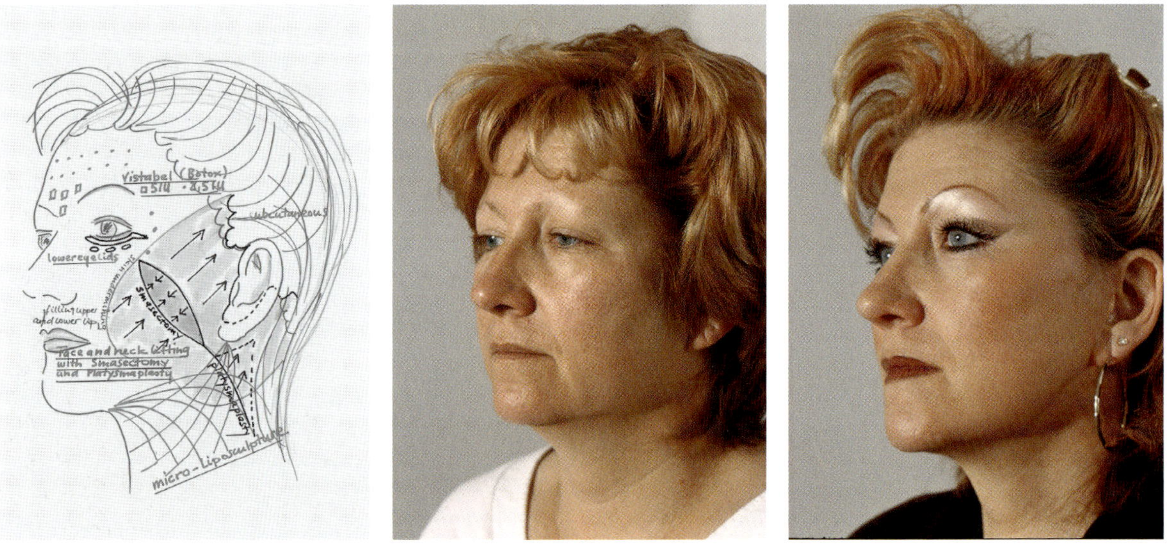

7 Face and neck lift with SMAS-ectomy, platysmaplasty and micro liposculpture, lower blepharoplasty, micro lipofilling of upper and lower lip, injection of Vistabel® (botulinum toxin) in frontal and outer orbital region

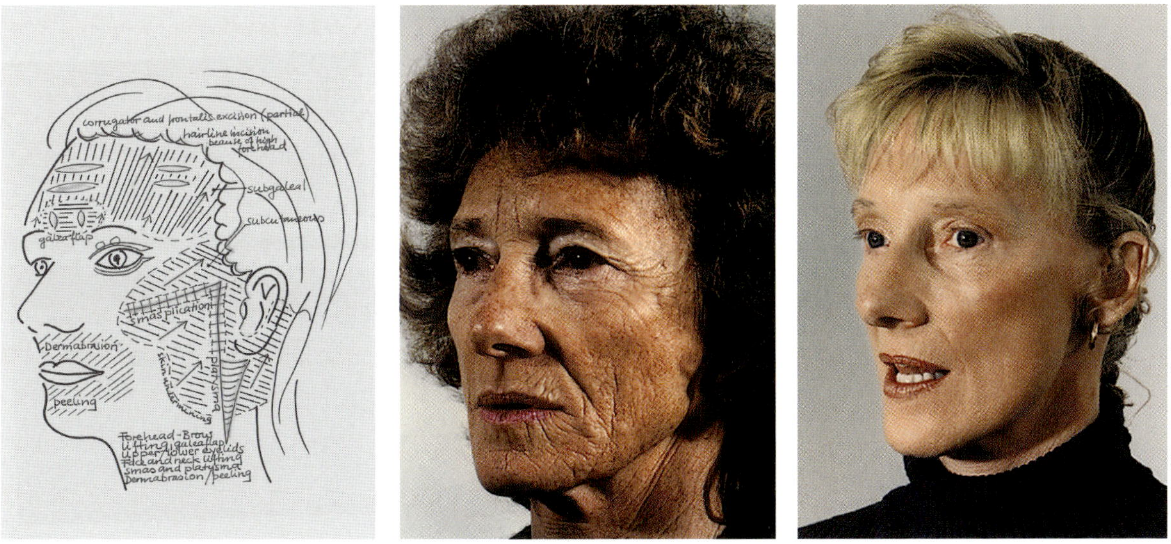

8 Forehead and eyebrow lift with myoplasties, face lift with SMAS-plication, neck lift with platysmaplasty, upper and lower blepharoplasty, dermabrasion of upper lip and peeling of lower lip

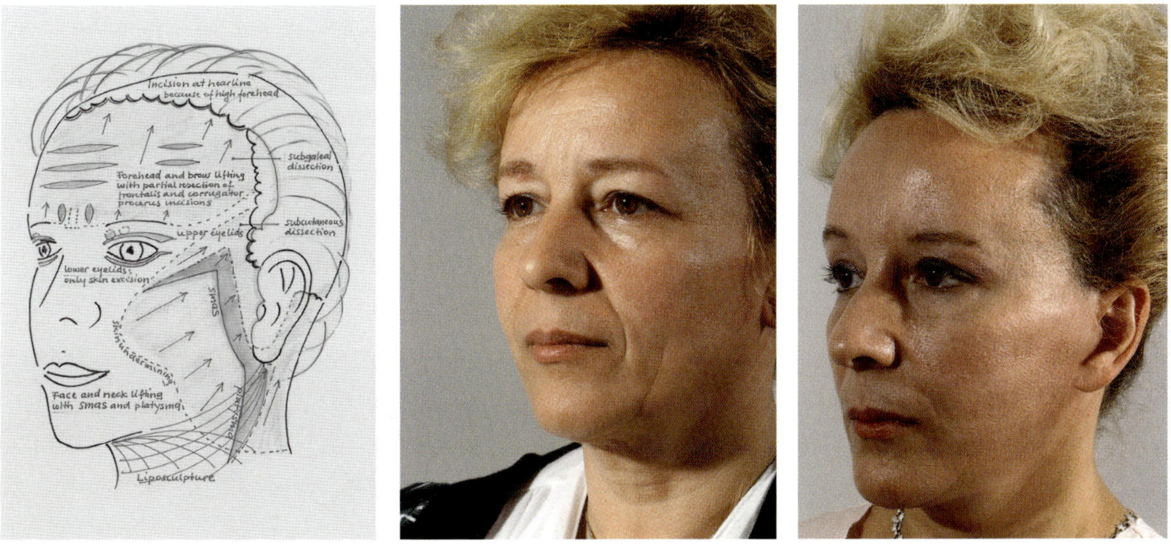

9 Forehead and eyebrow lift with myoplasties, face lift with SMAS, neck lift with platysmaplasty and micro liposculpture, upper and lower blepharoplasty

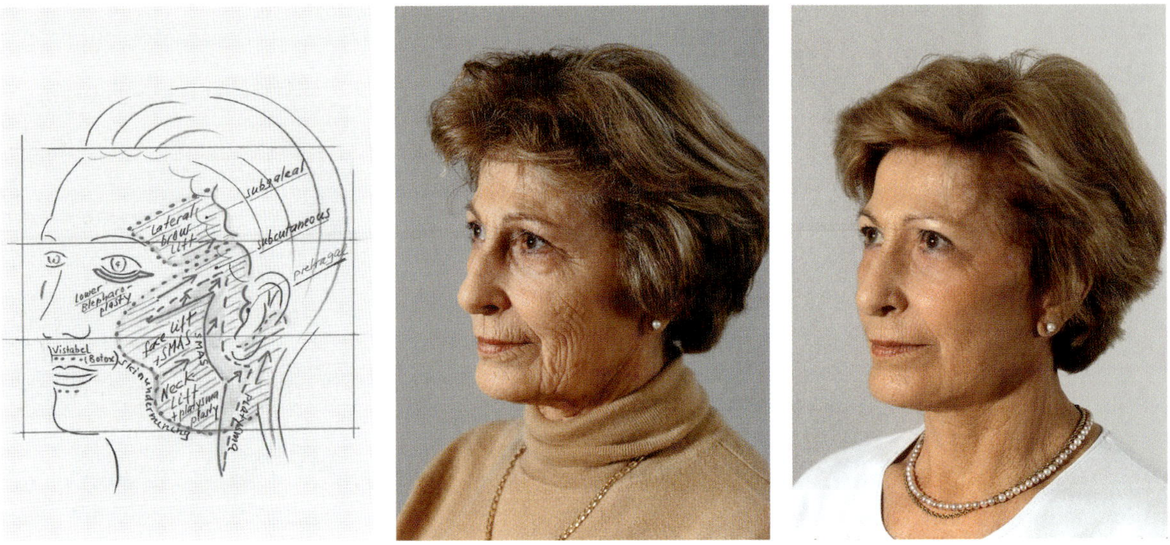

10 Temple lift, face and neck lift with SMAS and platysmaplasty, lower blepharoplasty, injections of Vistabel® (botulinum toxin) and hyaluronic acid in upper and lower lips

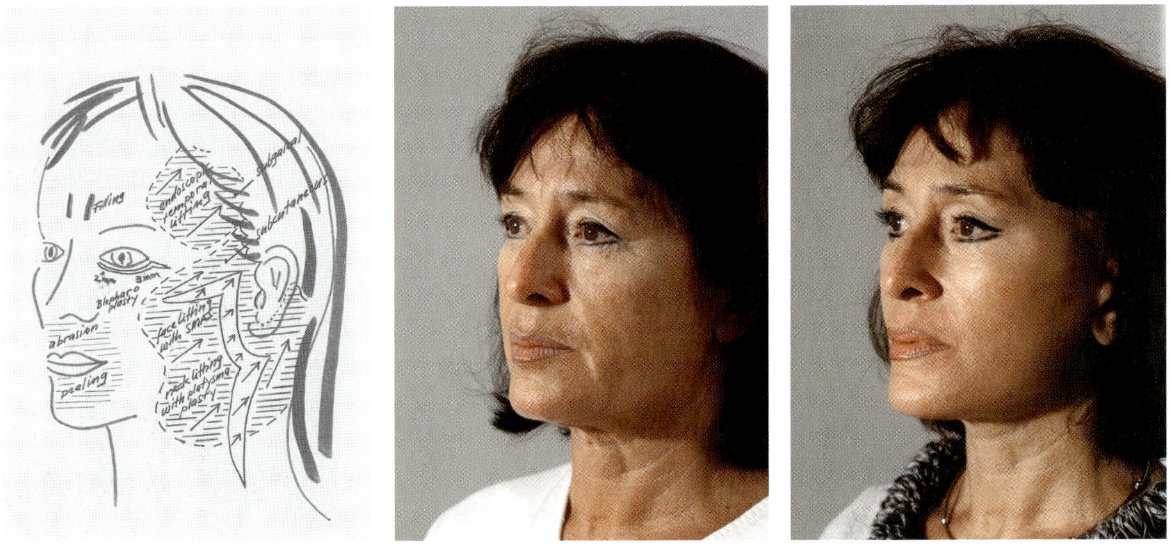

11 Endoscopic temple lift, face lift with SMAS, neck lift with platysmaplasty, lower blepharoplasty, filling of the frown lines, dermabrasion of upper lip, peeling of lower lip

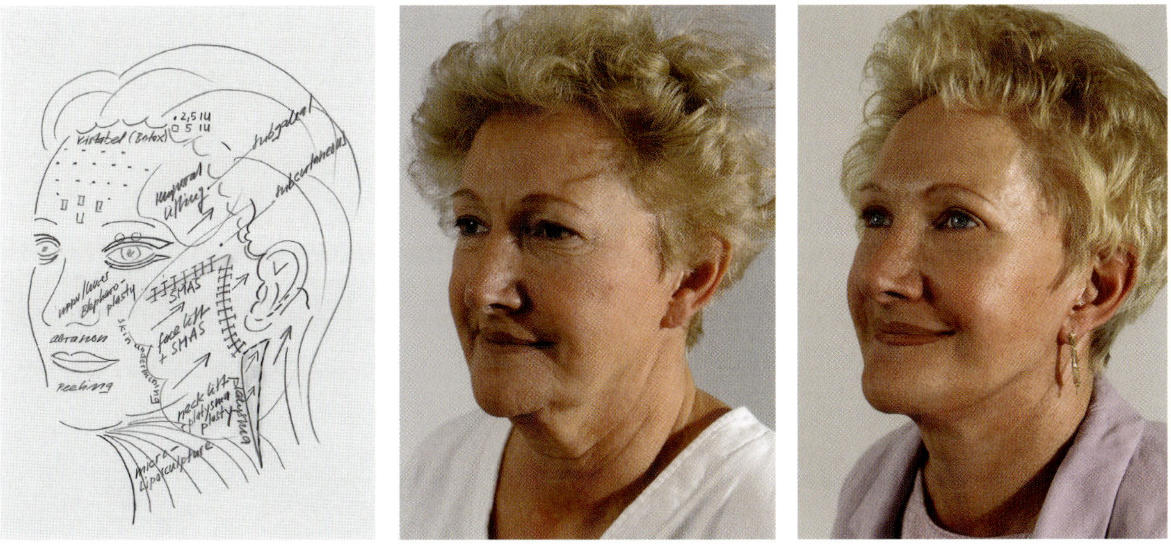

12 Endoscopic temple lift, face lift with SMAS, neck lift with platysmaplasty and micro liposculpture, upper and lower blepharoplasty, light dermabrasion of upper lip, peeling of lower lip, injections of Vistabel® (botulinum toxin) in forehead region

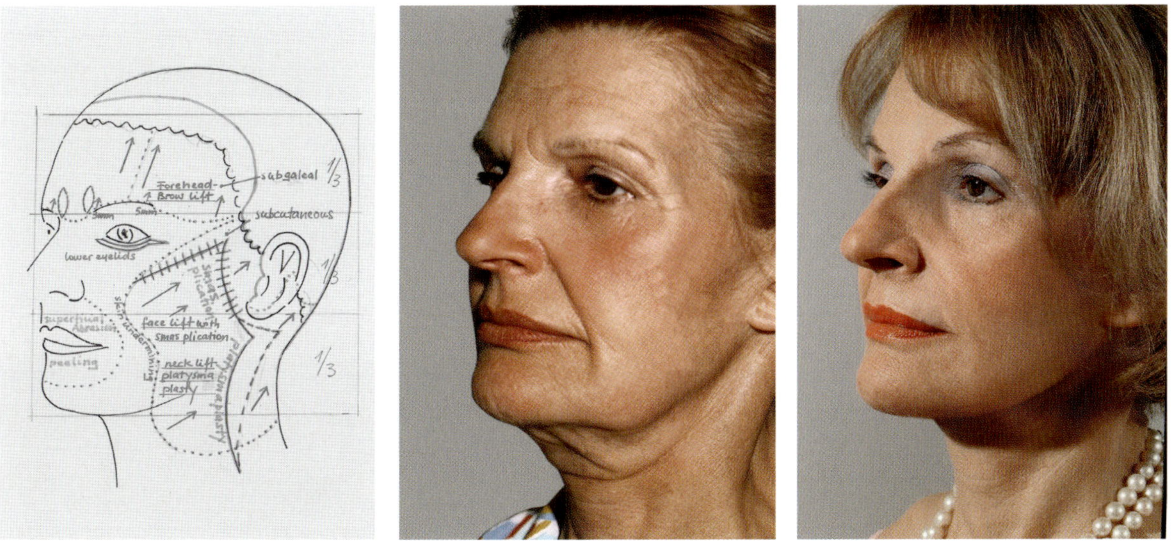

13 Forehead and eyebrow lift with myoplasties, face and neck lift with SMAS and platysmaplasty, lower blepharoplasty, dermabrasion of upper lip, peeling of lower lip

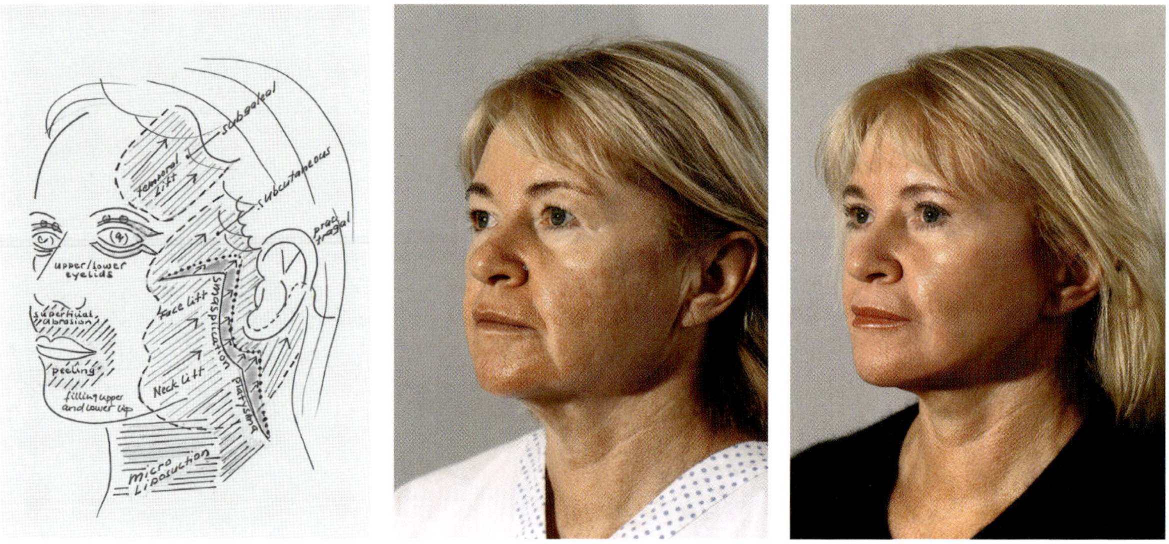

14 Temple lift, face lift with SMAS, neck lift with platysmaplasty and micro liposculpture, upper and lower blepharoplasty, light dermabrasion of upper lip, peeling of lower lip, micro lipofilling of upper and lower lip

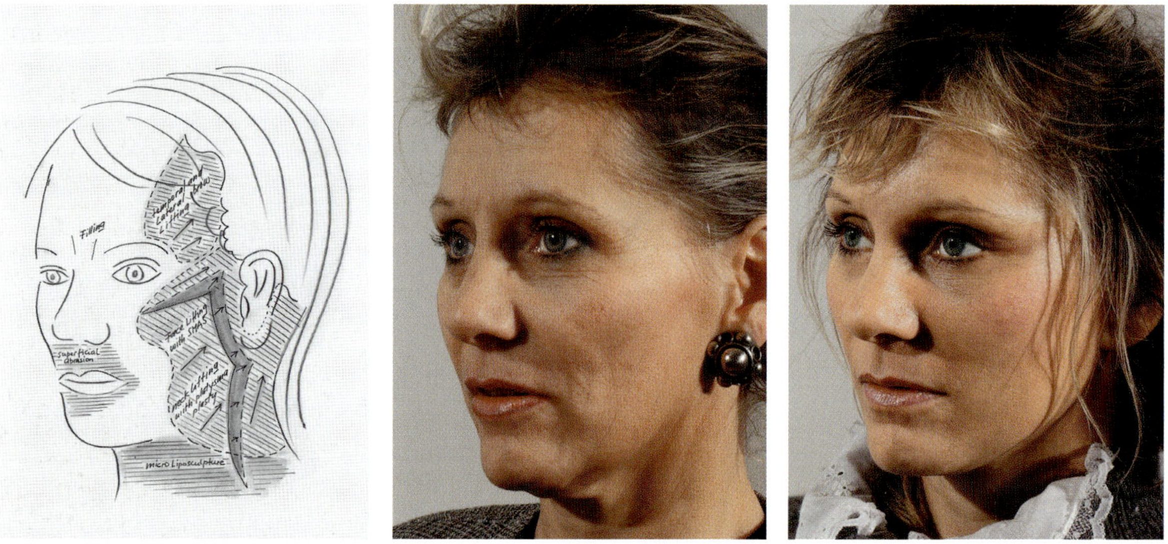

15 Temple lift, face lift with SMAS, neck lift with platysmaplasty and micro liposculpture, filling of frown lines, light dermabrasion of upper and lower lips

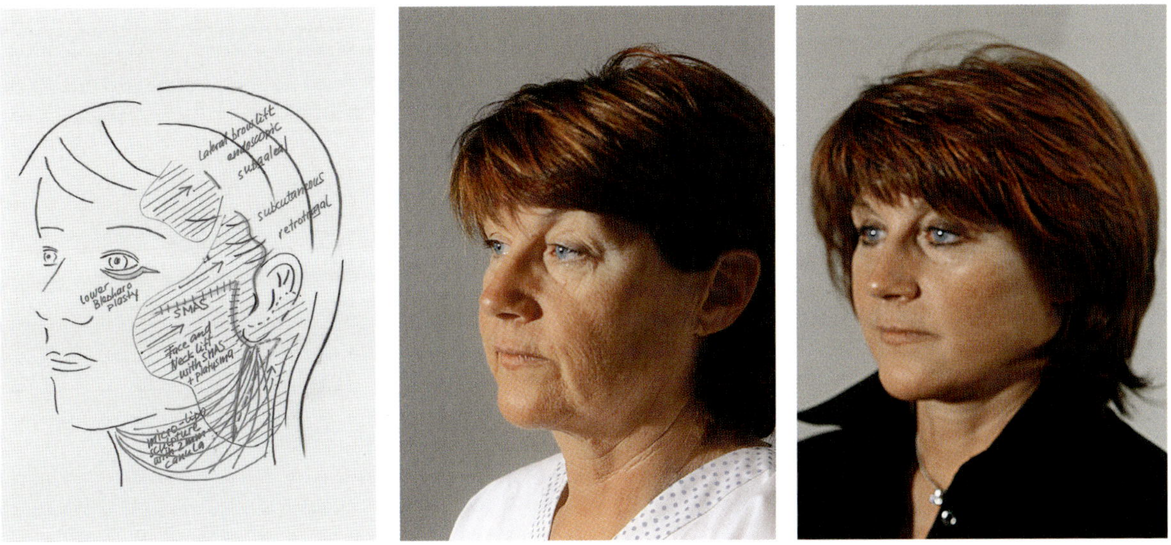

16 Endoscopic temple lift, face lift with SMAS, neck lift with platysmaplasty and micro liposculpture, lower blepharoplasty

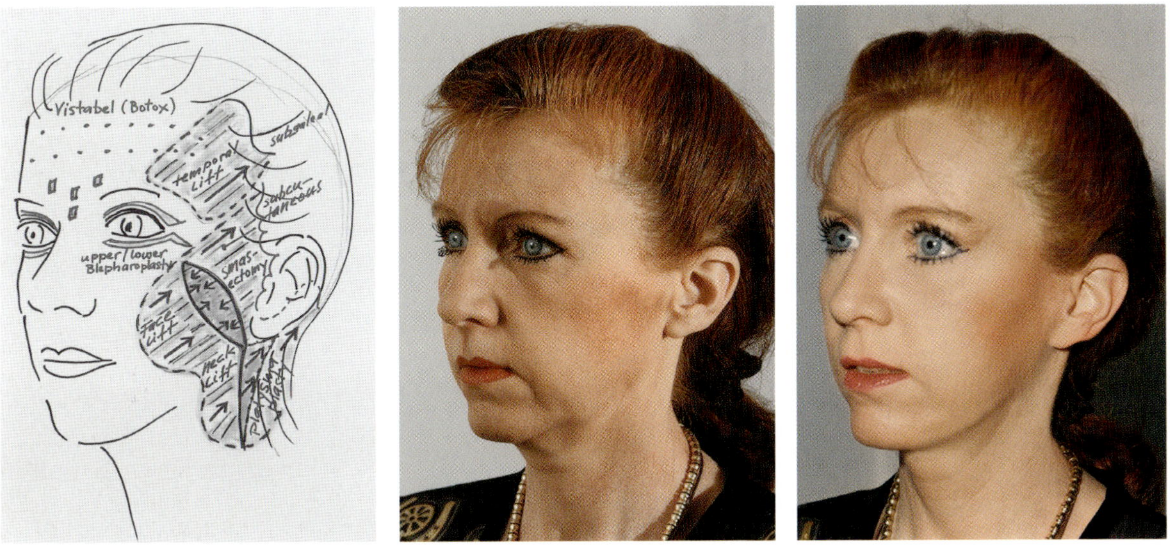

17 Temple lift, face and neck lift with SMAS-ectomy and platysmaplasty, upper and lower blepharoplasty, injections of Vistabel® (botulinum toxin) in forehead and outer orbital regions

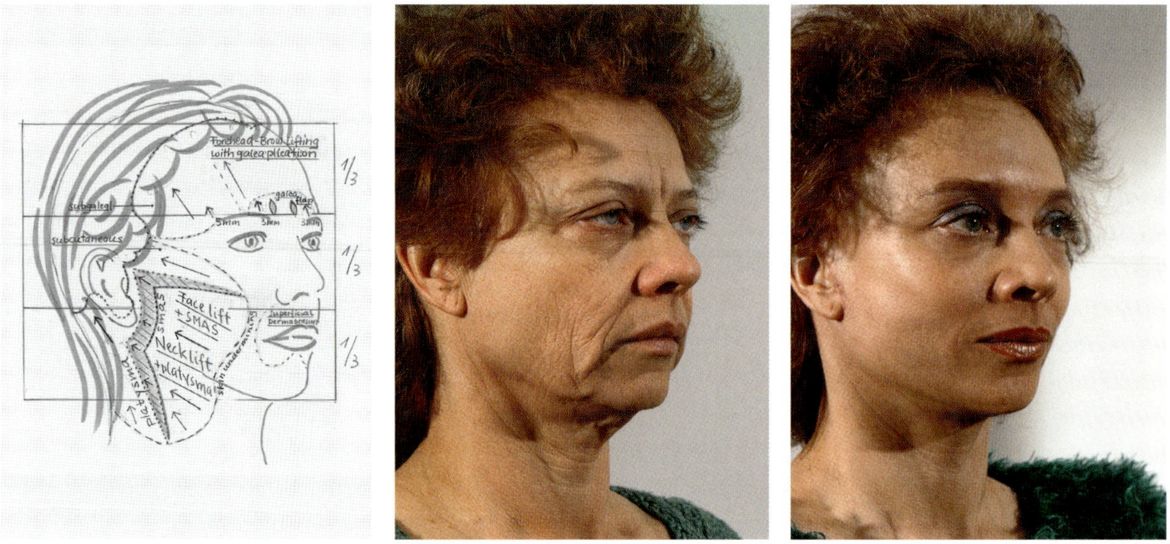

18 Forehead and eyebrow lift with myoplasties, face and neck lift with SMAS and platysmaplasty, superficial dermabrasion of upper and lower lips

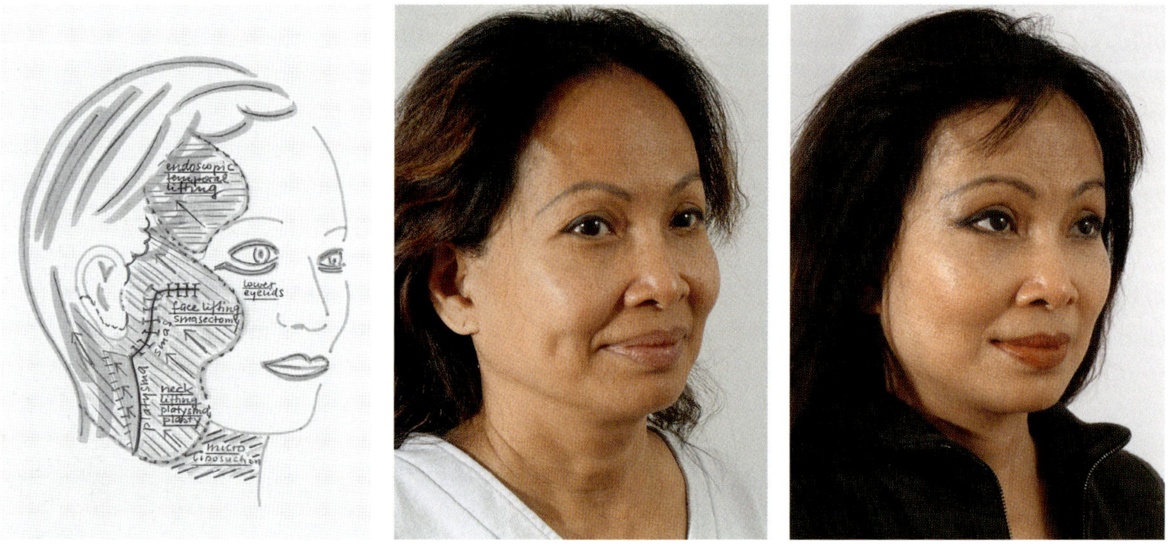

19 Endoscopic temple lift, face lift with SMAS-plication, neck lift with platysmaplasty and micro liposculpture, lower blepharoplasty

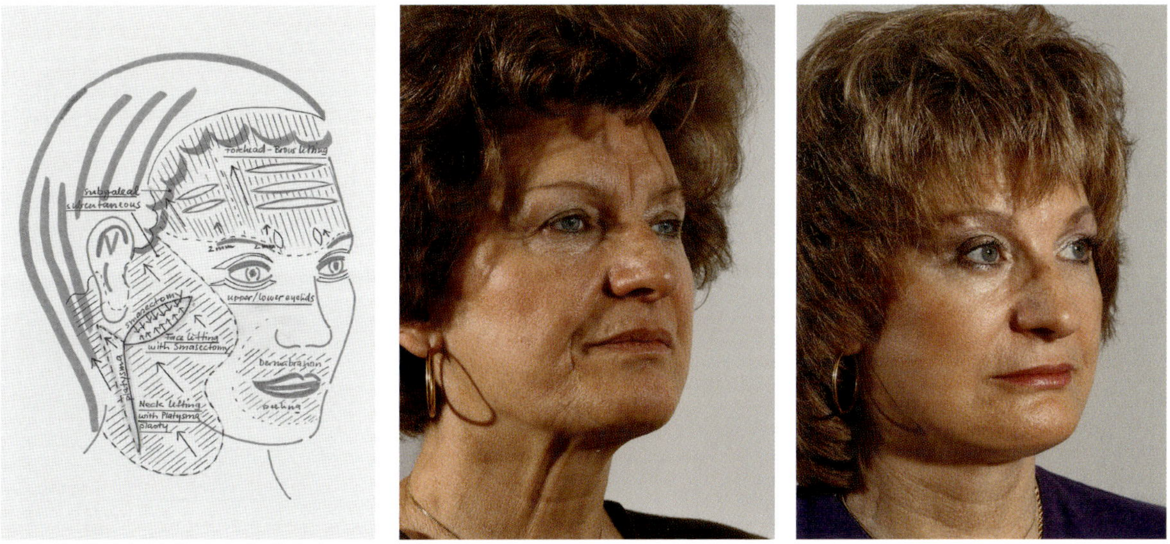

20 Forehead and eyebrow lift with myoplasties, face lift with SMAS-ectomy, neck lift with platysmaplasty, upper and lower blepharoplasty, dermabrasion of upper lip, peeling of lower lip

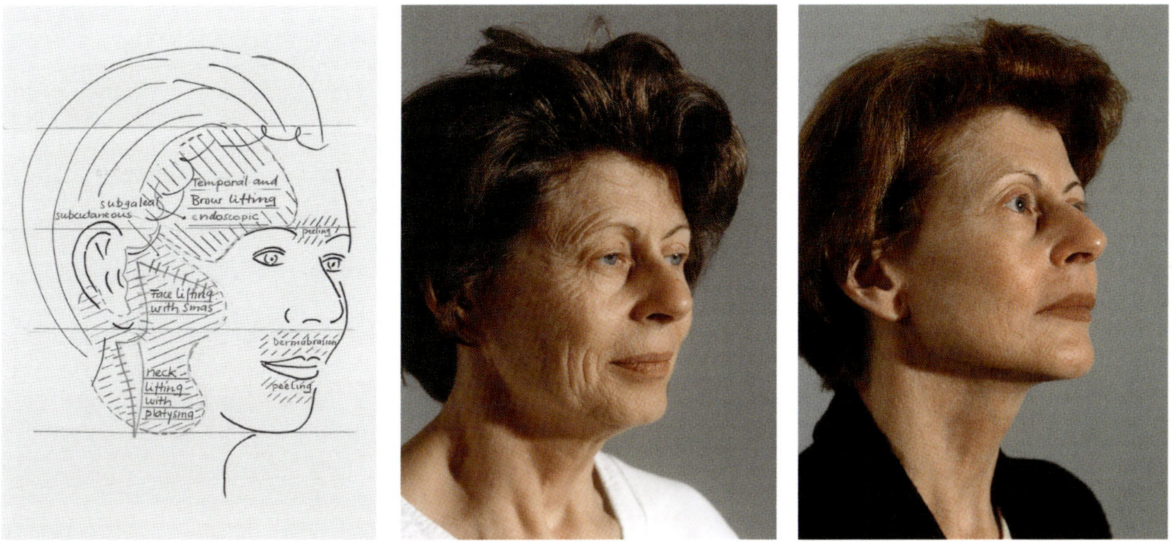

21 Endoscopic temple lift, face and neck lift with SMAS-plication and platysmaplasty, light dermabrasion of upper lip, peeling of the region between the brows and peeling of lower lip

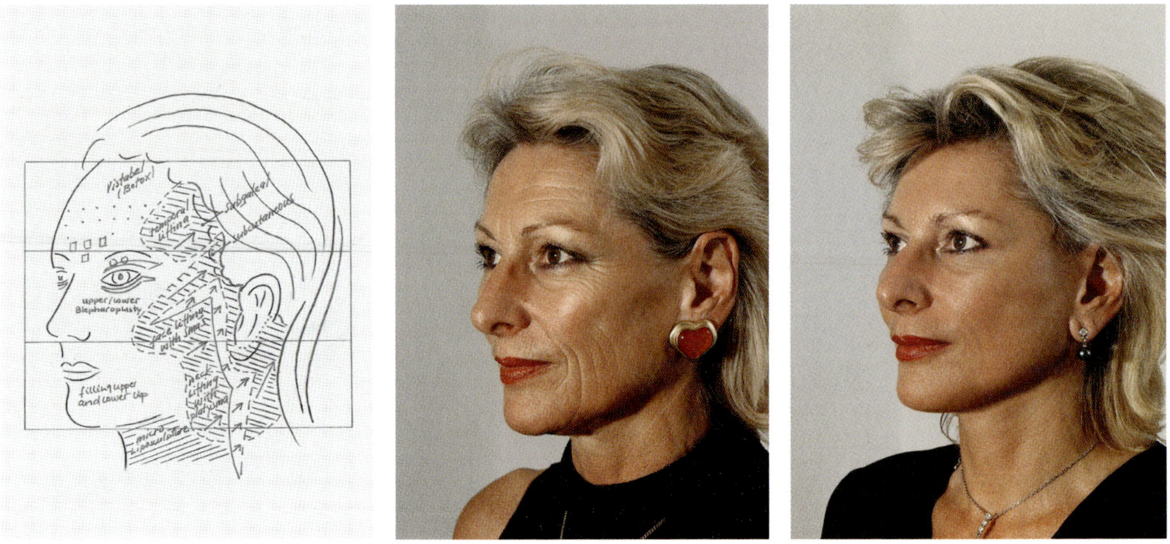

22 Temple lift, face lift with SMAS, neck lift with platysmaplasty and micro liposculpture, upper and lower blepharoplasty, micro lipofilling of upper and lower lip, injections of Vistabel® (botulinum toxin) in forehead and outer orbital regions

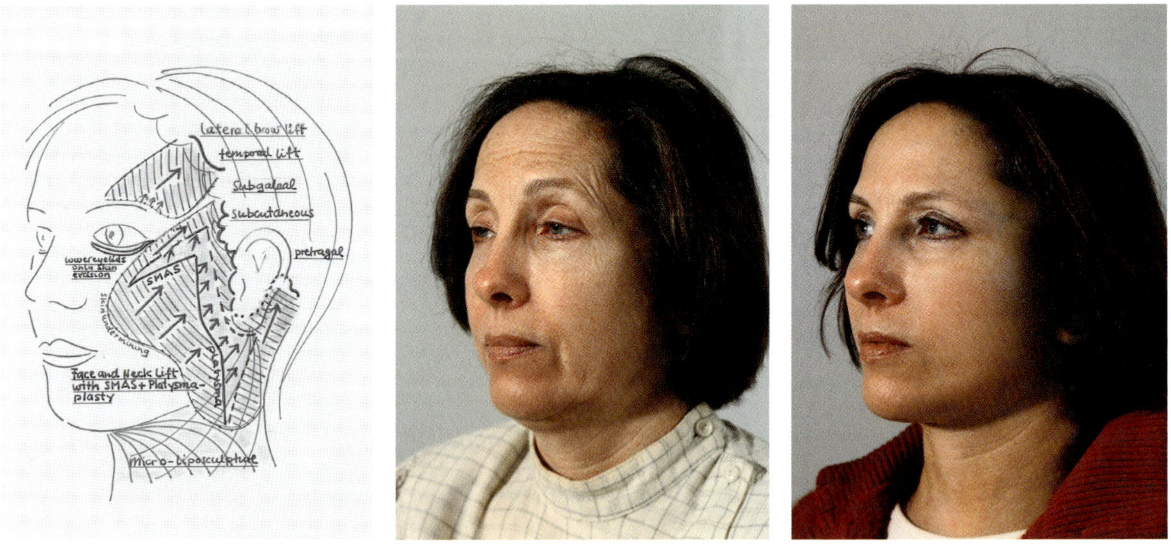

23 Temple lift, face lift with SMAS, neck lift with platysmaplasty and micro liposculpture, lower blepharoplasty

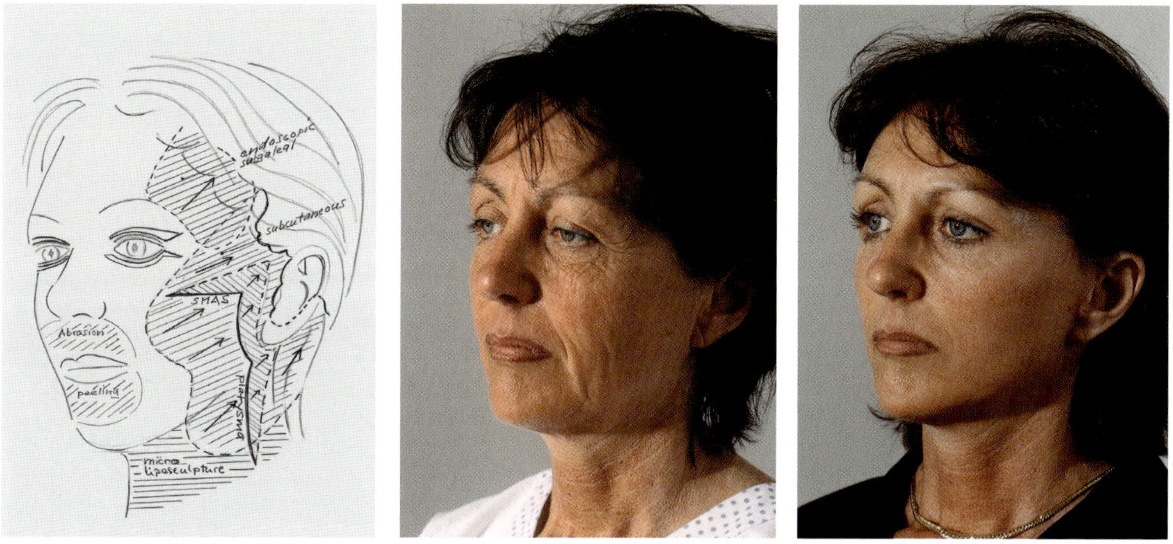

24 Endoscopic temple lift, face lift with SMAS, neck lift with platysmaplasty and micro liposculpture, upper and lower blepharoplasty, superficial dermabrasion of upper lip and peeling of lower lip, micro lipofilling of upper and lower lip

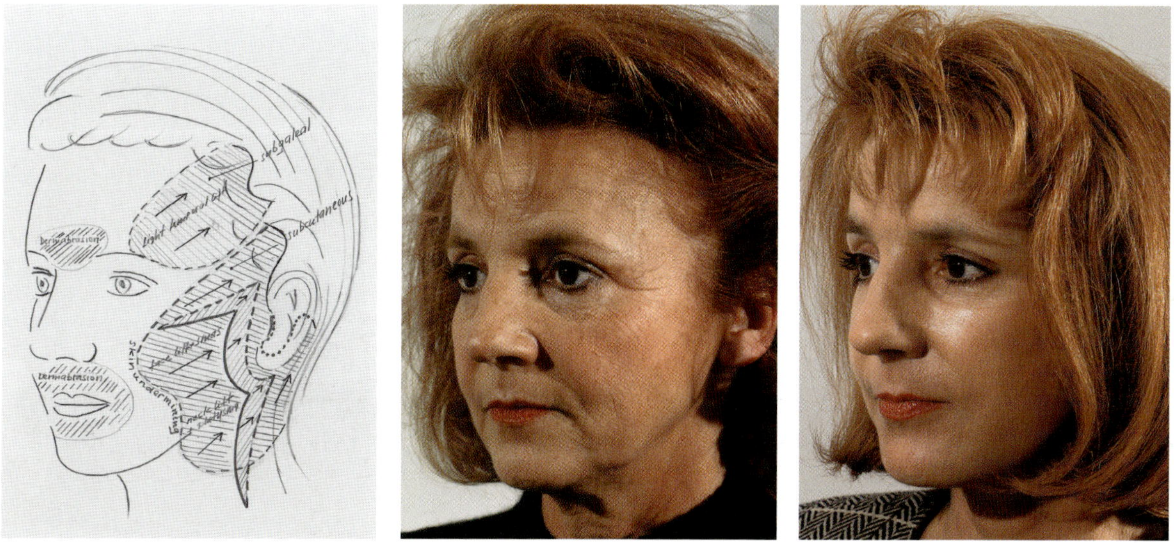

25 Light temple lift, face and neck lift with SMAS and platysmaplasty, dermabrasion of region between the brows and peeling of the upper and lower lips

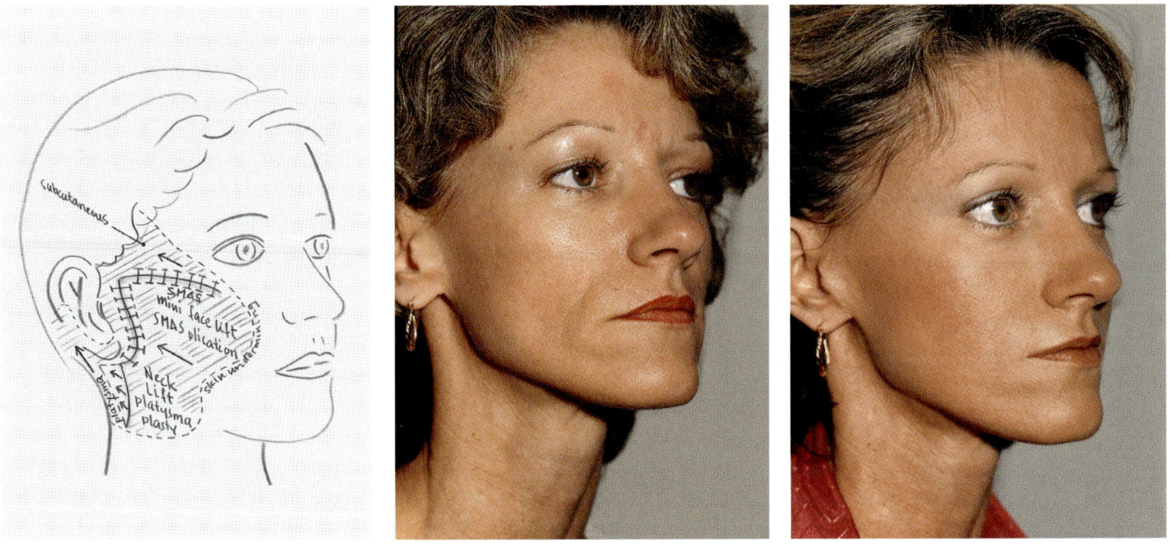

26 Mini-face lift with SMAS and platysmaplasty

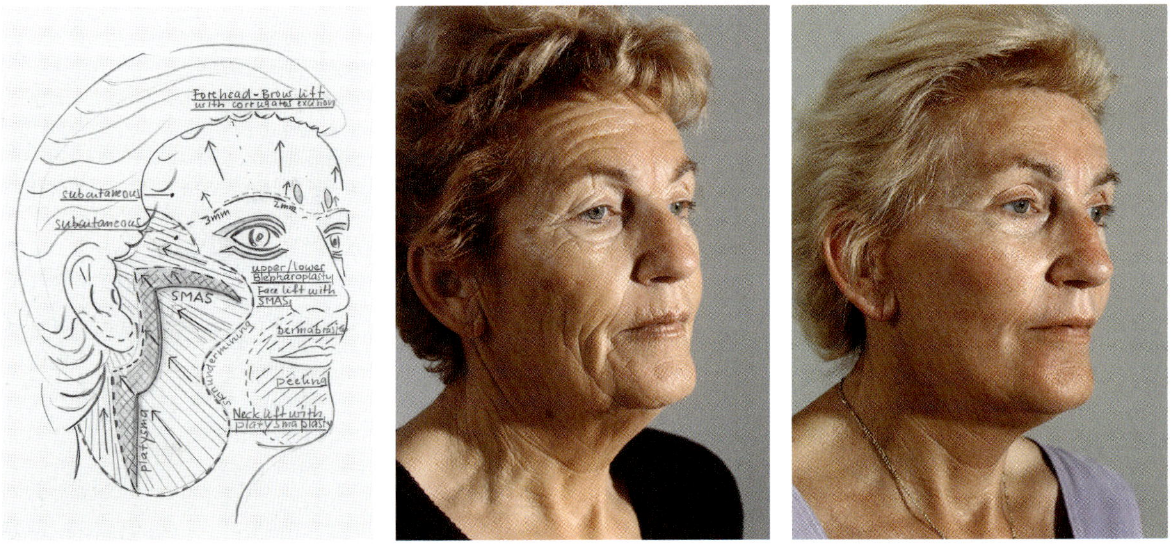

27 Forehead lift with myoplasties, face and neck lift with SMAS and platysmaplasty, upper and lower blepharoplasty, dermabrasion of upper lip, peeling of lower lip

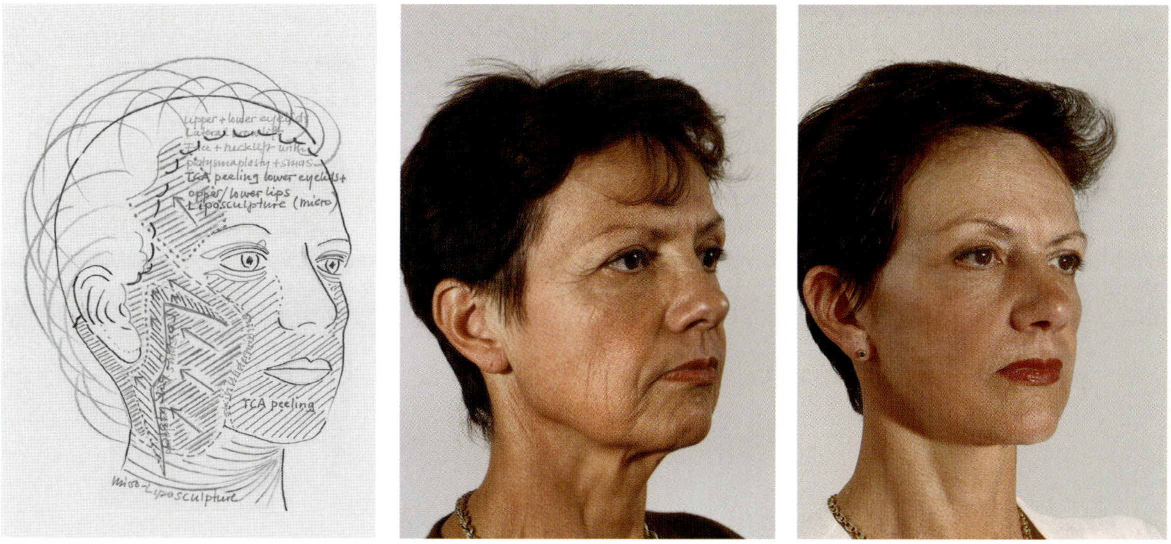

28 Temple lift, face lift with SMAS, neck lift with platysmaplasty and micro liposculpture, upper and lower blepharoplasty, peeling of lower eyelids and upper and lower lips

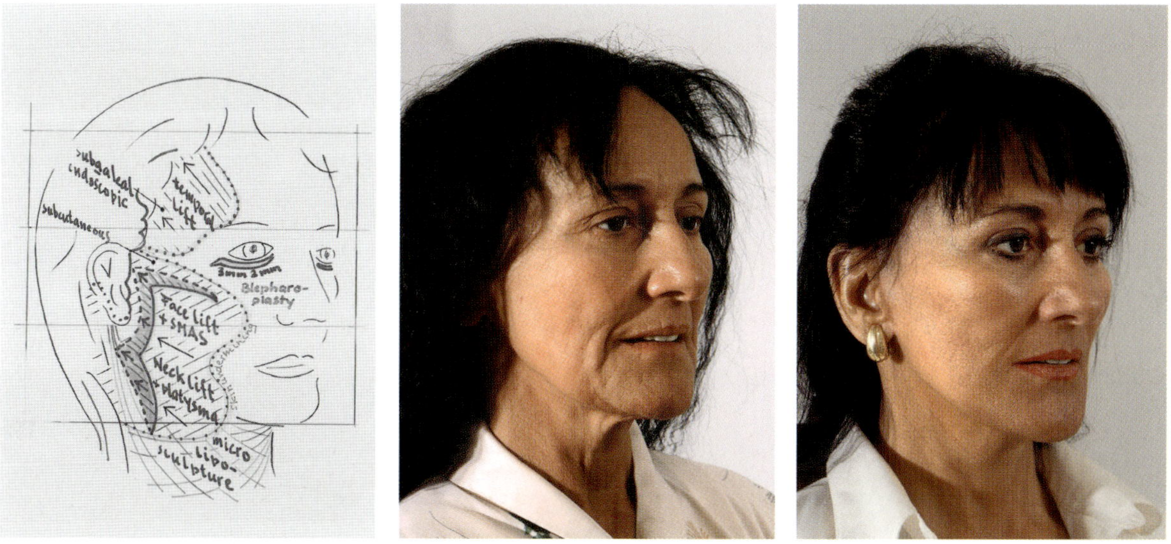

29 Endoscopic temple lift, face and neck lift with SMAS and platysmaplasty, lower blepharoplasty

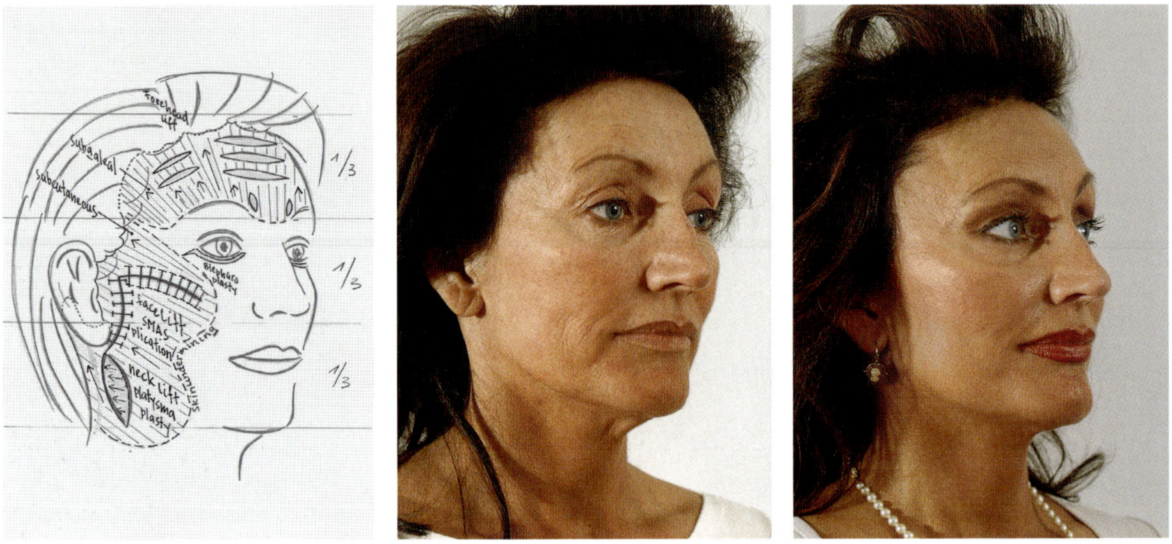

30 Forehead lift with myoplasties, face lift with SMAS-plication, neck lift with platysmaplasty, lower blepharoplasty

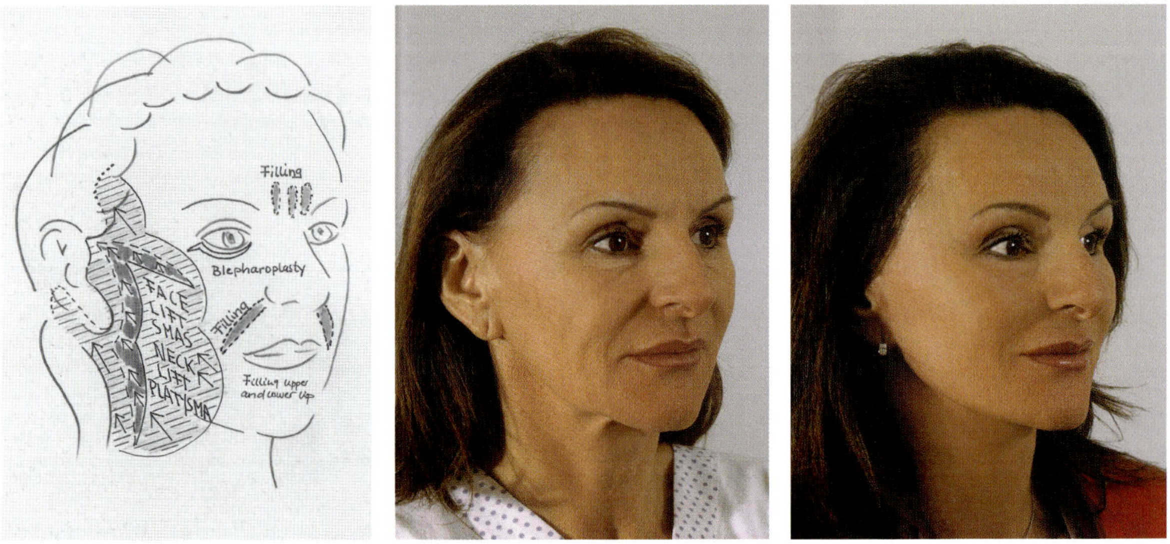

31 Face and neck lift with SMAS and platysmaplasty, micro lipofilling of the frown lines, the nasolabial folds and the upper and lower lip

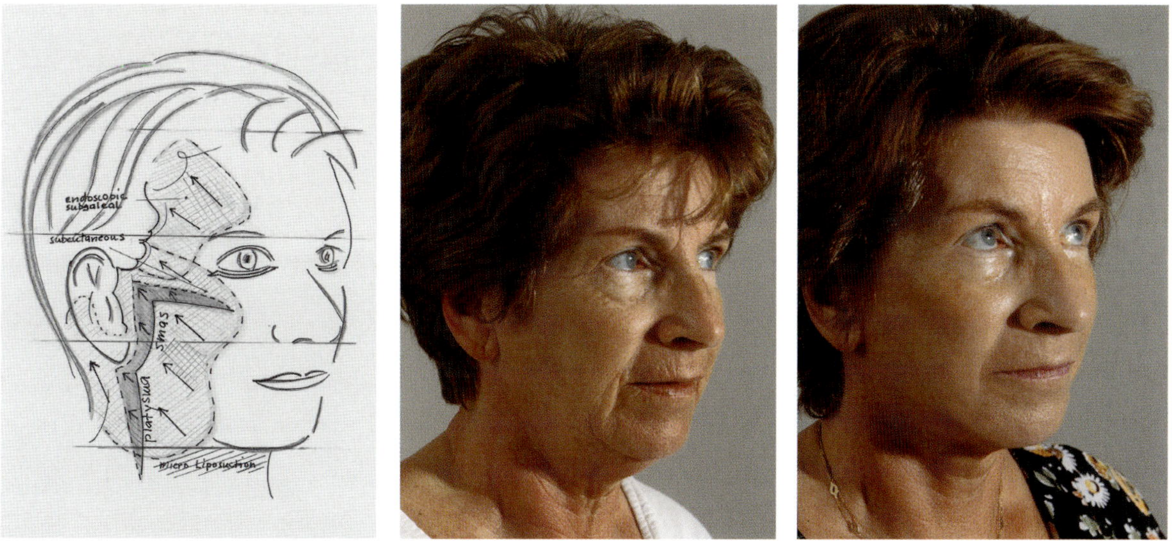

32 Endoscopic temple lift, face lift with SMAS, neck lift with platysmaplasty and micro liposculpture, lower blepharoplasty

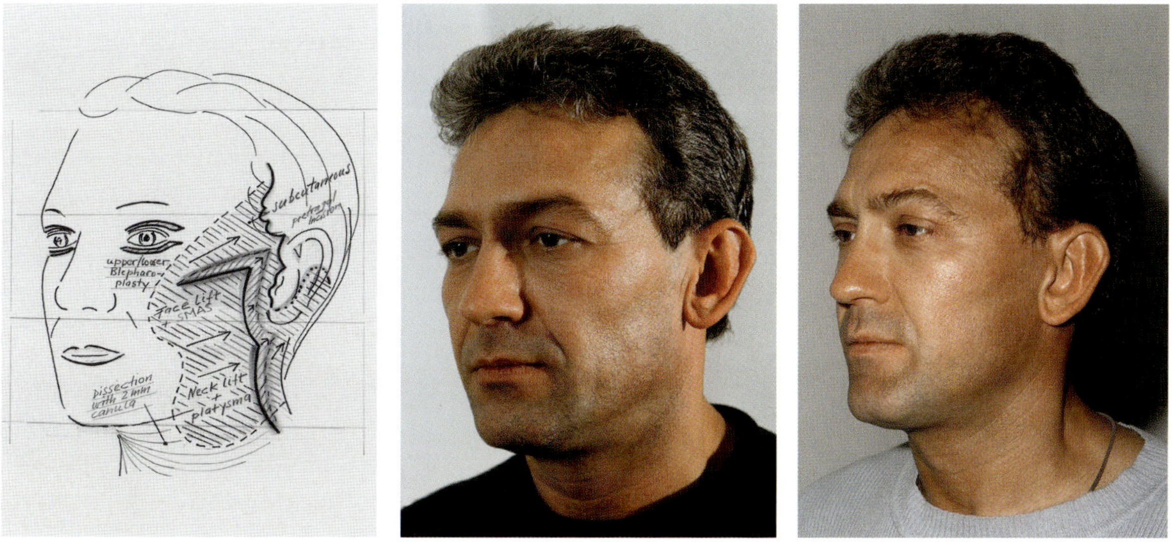

33 Face and necklift with SMAS and platysmaplasty, upper and lower blepharoplasty

Face Lift Patients Share Their Experience

Working in the stock-exchange department of a bank was much more than just a job for me. It was really my whole world. Like for many things in my life, I also had to fight for a long time to get this job. So I was happy and filled with a great sense of self-esteem because I had managed, on my own merit, to gain access to a world which fifteen years ago had been exclusively reserved for men. But the many hours of overtime and the hectic pace of daily life in the stock exchange department had – after a few years – also taken a lot out of me with the result that at age fourty-five I noticed a slightly tired expression and severe features in my face, which made me feel uneasy.

The fact that I used to pay attention in my life to my health and diet, as well as doing a sufficient amount of sport, contributed a lot to preserving my well-formed, slim body. I did not adopt this philosophy of life by chance, as my parents were very sporting and health-conscious. In my youth I practised ski racing together with my elder brother and took part in many international competitions. At the age of fifteen I gave up top-class sport and then worked as a ski instructor. When at the age of thirty I met the man who was to become my partner – a former professional cyclist, but who at the time was the director and sporting manager of his own successful team of professional cyclists – I began to take an interest in cycle racing. I used to accompany him regularly in my leisure time to the national and international cycle races and also began to cycle myself. As a keen sports cyclist I myself used to ride four to five thousand kilometres a year on my racing bike – and still do so today although I'm now sixty years old. I was a confidante to the young, highly-trained athletes, listening to their worries and problems, encouraging them to produce their maximum performance and comforting them.

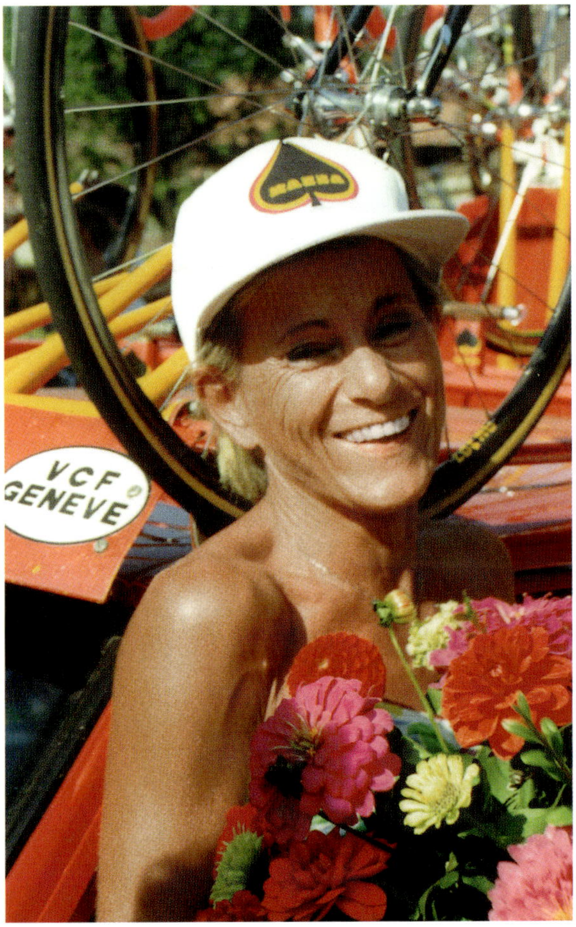

Eliane Guichard

My face had clearly grown older with the years. When I was fourty-eight I decided to have a face lift. In keeping with my temperament, I wanted to have the operation done immediately. I had known Dr. Urs Burki for a long time. He had already proven his great ability in the field of aesthetic surgery on some of my girlfriends. So I had great confidence in him. The result of the operation exceeded all my expectations! Only a few days after the intervention I already looked as I had at the age of thirty-five. I would never have thought such a thing was possible. My facial features had not been changed at all by the operation; I had been rejuvenated, but only in an extremely harmonious and natural way. When I look today at photos that were taken in the years prior to my operation, I can hardly imagine I had such a tired facial expression at that time. It's surprising how quickly one gets accustomed to one's new face.

It did not matter to me that my partner was not very supportive of my decision to have a face lift. The fact is that he was so enthusiastic about my very successful rejuvenation that he decided to have a minor nose correction performed on himself. Are we women not often the secret pioneers for decisions that men believe they are taking on their own?

Mrs. Eliane Guichard, Beaucaire, France

I've always been passionately keen on sports. Sport forms an extremely pleasant counterbalance to my professional activity. I very often practise sports with young people, whose zest for a challenge I share. Water skiing and surfing are my favourite water sports. When I play golf – which is usually frustrating for a perfectionist – I try to remain positive and restrain my temperament, but also to train my concentration and coordination of movement sequences. In winter, on the other hand, I feel an urge to go up into the mountains, where as an enthusiastic snowboarder I would most of all like to leave my tracks in the soft powdery snow far off the prepared ski slopes – but for safety reasons I keep to the marked ski runs. Fitness is part of my personal timetable three times a week. Physical fitness to me is in harmony with intellectual performance – *mens sana in corpore sano*.

What makes my profession so attractive? Its diversity. It's a fascinating discipline that brings you face to face daily with many different aspects of life and requires me to deal with multi-faceted human problems. There's no routine, but a constant attention to detail. It's a magnificent profession which enables you to establish many rich and varied contacts, but a very demanding, even pitiless job, in which external appearances make or mark the first contact with both the client and the judge. The profession of lawyer is a job in which a person's facial expression and physique help to determine whether or not the indispensable relationship of trust is established.

There's nothing superficial about aestheticism or the pursuit of beauty. For my part, I consider that aesthetics extends well beyond the concept of beauty. Aesthetic sensitivity goes hand in hand with order, cleanliness and respect for oneself and other people. Taking care of one's person is also a sign of consideration for others. Paying attention to aesthetics is a way of life and an attitude of mind that also encompasses caring for and strengthening the body, a refinement that was already highly-developed by the Ancient Greeks.

Being satisfied with my physique, I would most probably never have thought of a face lift if I hadn't sustained a very serious cycling accident a few years ago. It was the desire to correct the scar on my forehead and the resultant slight asymmetry at the level of the superciliary arch that made me turn to aesthetic surgery and more specifically to Dr. Urs Burki, after having consulted several other plastic surgeons who were unable to convince me. Having grown up in a family of entrepreneurs and architects, I'm very sensitive to correct proportions and the harmony that emanates from them. The face has something special that touches on our innermost self. I had already consulted several plastic surgeons. The aesthetic correction I wanted to obtain didn't seem easy to achieve. A sur-

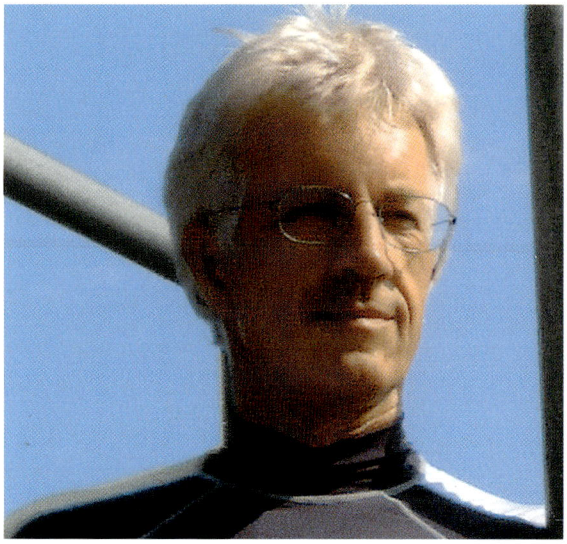

Bernhard Cron

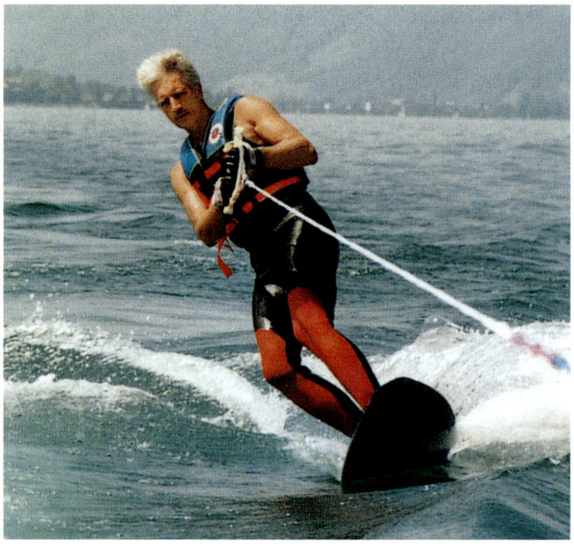

geon who had examined me intimated that the accident had made me look ten years older. Today, with a successful face lift, I've redeemed those years.

When I first met Dr. Burki, I liked several things about him right away. First of all, the fact that he's able to judge a situation quickly because he has so many references and comparisons, which denotes sound expertise, the result of experience. Then, an ability to make an accurate assessment and use clear language. After he had first listened to me carefully, Dr. Burki explained the planned operating procedure clearly and comprehensively, in all details. The scar from the face lift would be located not at the hairline since I do a lot of sport, which pushes my hair backwards and would make the scar more visible, but in a natural fold of the forehead, which would also attenuate the scar from the accident. I liked the idea right away. Another important point was that the operation didn't require general anaesthesia. But above all, with Dr. Burki I was sure he would do only what would contribute to a natural and harmonious result. It was also very important for me to be assured that my natural facial features would be kept unaltered.

I was convinced that the operation would be a success, because I was in excellent health, physically and mentally fit and knew that with Dr. Burki I was in the hands of a master of his art. But what I hadn't foreseen was that my professional activities would catch up with me again so quickly. I had been waiting for a judgement to be handed down for a long time. It came on the day of the operation. I had ten days to finalize a notice of appeal. The evening of the operation my secretary brought me the file, which I began to work on immediately and the next day I went back to the office. On top of this there was already a family celebration coming up at the weekend.

Really very happy with my face lift, about six months later I spent an evening with a charming young lady who noticed nothing about the operation and, what is more, thought I was ten years younger. Sixteen months have gone by since then and our marriage and the birth of Alexander are imminent.

Mr. Bernhard Cron, Geneva

Although I try to keep to a healthy diet, I am by no means averse to culinary delights. I'm a gourmet who loves tasting delicious dishes in exclusive restaurants. Sport (tennis, windsurfing, swimming, skating, cross-country skiing, mountain hiking and biking, jogging competitions including the famous Morat-Fribourg marathon) is an important part of my healthy, well-balanced lifestyle.

As for many women, one day the time came when I began to draw back the skin on my cheeks as I looked at myself in the mirror. I just couldn't believe that the skin of my face had become so sagging. One day my husband said to me: "It's crazy, but your face doesn't match your body at all". I felt like a wreck, but nevertheless he was perfectly right. My face had indeed aged prematurely in comparison to my body.

Until then, I had never been interested in aesthetic surgery. Why should I? I like everything the natural way, especially where my body is concerned. Wrinkles don't bother me. I've accepted ageing. But I wanted this ageing process to be harmonious and above all, my face to correspond to my age and athletic body. However, having an operation on one's face is not a decision to be taken lightly.

Until now, I have not regretted for one single moment my decision. I'm not a pin-up, but the way I look now is sufficient to feel at ease with myself. That's the main thing. I adopted my new image right away especially because it looked so natural.

I have done a lot of walks with my dog, and my face healed very quickly. I'm convinced that eighty per cent of the people who saw me two weeks later didn't notice anything. They simply thought I was looking good and the many compliments I received were like balsam for my soul. When I went back to work two weeks later, I didn't want to talk about the operation, not out of shame - especially as I now had the face I'd always dreamt of having and which suits me perfectly - but rather out of pride and a woman's natural concern for her appearance.

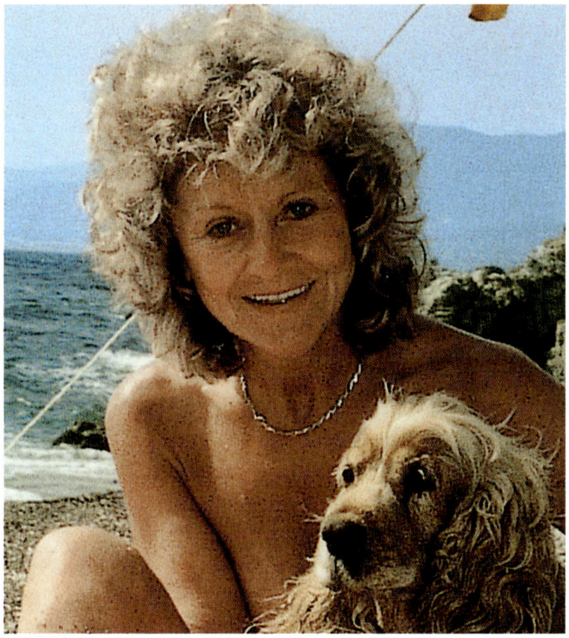

Erika André

I realize that the operation changes us deep below the skin as well. It is not just the appearance but the well-being that we radiate when everything's been a success. It is not so much the way other people look at me; it is me who's changed in my relationship with other people. I've got more self-confidence. I find it easier to look people straight in the face. Previously, if they held my gaze, I gradually began to feel uncomfortable at the idea they were going to see my wrinkles and jowls. As a result of the operation I have become generally more self-assured, an advantage which I appreciate, especially at business meetings.

Who knows, I may never have taken the decision to have a face lift, if my husband, an artist-painter, sportsman and *bon vivant* who is deeply attached to nature, hadn't made such a pertinent remark about my face...

Mrs. Erika André, Saint-Cergue (Switzerland)

When I was young, I was adored, famous, a star in my own right. I was popular, looked attractive and was successful in my work, which I loved more than anything else, because I was able to make full use of my creativity and fulfil my strong need to communicate and to share. In fact, I had everything I needed to be happy...

And still, I had never experienced in full the happiness of being a beautiful woman. Even though I was expecting men to appreciate my beauty, I myself didn't really acknowledge it. I had gradually seen my face change as my ideas and feelings changed, and I'd seen my features being moulded by what I was thinking and experiencing. I realized that I was in the process of losing something that was essential for me. One day I noticed that my face bore the marks of great sadness.

It was for myself that I was having the face lift done. It was something that came from within rather than from an external influence. It wasn't so much the idea of being rejuvenated or looking more beautiful that was the motivation for my face lift. It was rather the desire to make my physiognomy match my actual happy feelings. I wanted the expression on my face to correspond to what I was experiencing; in fact, I was in the process of rediscovering life!

I had consulted some women friends, but I wasn't particularly convinced about aesthetic surgery. Then I met Dr. Burki and my decision was made. I could tell from the way he examined me that it wasn't particularly the wrinkles he was observing, but that he imagined already how his work would release what was preventing the beauty of my face from revealing itself. What a magnificent result! Now I can age in beauty.

Mrs. Françoise Schaller, Cannes (France)

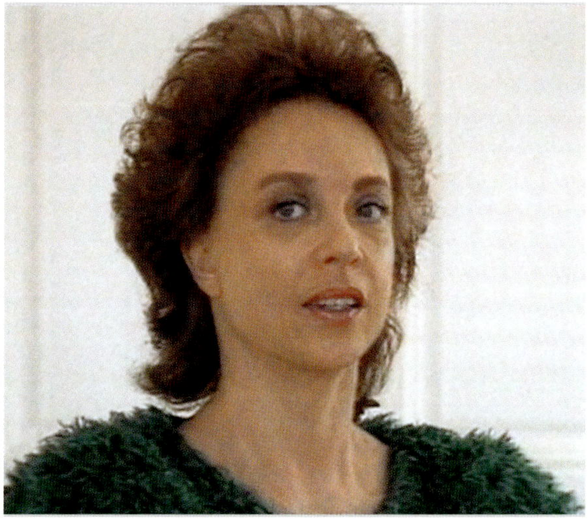

Françoise Schaller

Undergoing an operation is not a decision to be taken lightly. My experience was a very intense one. After some painful tribulations, of the type that bruise the soul, I had neglected myself somewhat. Can you imagine, going up from size 38 to 52, for someone like me who, as the owner of an elegant fashion boutique, had spent many years dressing other women? I could no longer find garments to fit me. Also, I was no longer this dynamic, sparkling lady who was so full of life. I couldn't go on like this! So I got things under control and solved first of all my weight problem.

One bright summer's day I met the woman who had been a witness at my wedding. As she hadn't seen me for a while, she thought I had aged a great deal. Without hesitating, she said to me: "Why don't you go and see an aesthetic surgeon?" The idea of entrusting myself to a surgeon's hands wasn't easy to swallow ... and how should I choose one in the first place? My girlfriend, who has been managing the famous Beauty Care Centre of the Grand Hotel in Evian-les-Bains for many years, told me to see Dr. Burki in Geneva. She said: "I've seen so many excellent results in customers who've had a facial rejuvenation operation performed by this surgeon that I'm totally convinced about his work. He's a magician!" Of course, after thirty years in the fashion trade, I've seen people who've had face lifts ... some of them were not very natural and harmonious. If I was to have a face lift, it shouldn't look like an operation being done, more like having been on a long holiday. I wanted to know more about the work of Dr. Burki and met a few women on whom he had performed a face lift. It was splendid work. Nothing could have convinced me more than these extraordinary results.

During the first consultation with Dr. Burki at his beautiful private Clinic, I immediately gained confidence in him. The confidence one has in one's surgeon is an essential part of the patient-doctor relationship. He said to me: "Mrs. Rolli, you're a woman who is brimming with energy, and that's what your face should reflect." Dr. Burki handed me some extensive documentation which enabled me to prepare for the operation, to ask him further questions during the next consultation so as to understand fully the solutions suggested by him and designed to restore the harmony of my face.

The operation was a fresh start in my life, a genuine rebirth which would never have been possible without this superb face lift. I regained my *joie de vivre* and my optimism. I can once again marvel at little things and enjoy life again to the full. For me, it's very important to admit openly that I have had a face lift. How else should I answer the question that I was asked time and time again: "But what have you done, Maité? You look splendid." One day I was contacted by a journalist from a Geneva daily. He wanted me to report on my face lift. I took this opportunity without hesitation and with great joy, because I felt the need to share my experiences with as many women as possible and to give courage to all those who were afraid of an aesthetic operation for some reason or another. I was concerned to tell the future patients how important it is to go to an experienced, well-trained aesthetic surgeon.

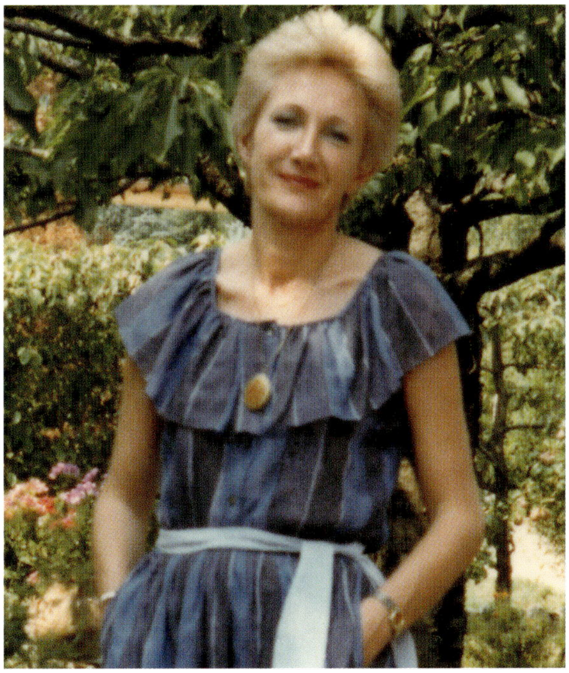

Marie-Thérèse Rolli

Ultimately, the success of an aesthetic operation depends entirely on him. Exchanging your personal experiences with other people gives you strength and also reinforces your self-esteem and self-confidence.

When I had the honour of being invited to attend the face lift Dr. Burki was performing in a concert hall in the presence of TV cameras, I went and sat in the front row straight away because it doesn't bother me if people know. Many friends and relatives and even some doctors phoned me afterwards because they'd seen me on TV and wanted to know more.

It's a pity I didn't have the idea of arranging for the operation to be performed in the open air. I would have loved to look up at the soothing blue of the sky during my rejuvenation surgery, breathed the sweet scent of the flowers and listened to the twittering of the birds and the trickling of the water ... What a great experience!

Mrs. Marie-Thérèse Rolli, Evian (France)

My native canton of Fribourg has given me an irrepressible love of nature and the mountains. I worked for a while as a journalist before going into paediatrics, where I took up an offer to be trained as an instrument operator. I liked this prospect, but after five years I had to make a choice; working at the weekends was getting me down. The call of the mountains triumphed. Finally, I found a job that enabled me to live out my passion. As a woman member of a fairly select mountain climbing club, I have always been able to take good care of myself; that's my great strength. As a regular roped party leader, I derive my sparkling energy from such magical places as the Matterhorn, Mont Blanc, in the Gastlosen; Aiguille du Plan, Dent du Géant, Les Dômes de Marge, not forgetting the Salève, where I frequently accompany elderly mountain climbing friends out of solidarity (the eldest is 92 years old!).

But the frequent exposure of my redhead's skin to the intensive sun of high mountains caused my face to age prematurely so that one day my daughter said to me: "You know, mum, you're getting terribly wrinkled." That triggered something in my mind. I thought it over and looked carefully at myself in the mirror. Indeed, the face I saw didn't reflect my overall youthfulness.

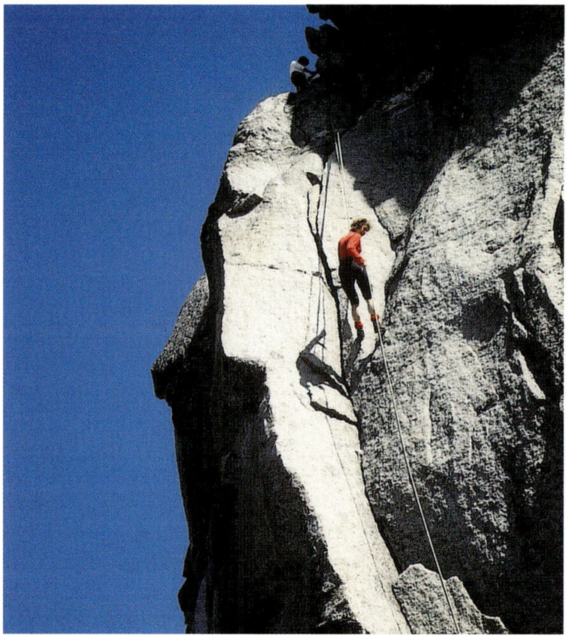

Climbing on the Grand Charmoz-Grepon, 3463 m

A relationship of trust was built with Dr. Burki straight away. Dr. Burki is an extraordinary surgeon because he doesn't alter the expression on your face. I would say it's even more than that: it's a rediscovery. You experience yourself differently. Before I was very shy. Today it's a pleasure for me to go out to the cinema, to the theatre and opera, to the restaurant. So I have gained a lot of self-confidence since my face lift.

And the operation? Everything was done in an atmosphere of harmony and I felt like going ahead in total security. A painless intervention, it was like lying on cotton wool, and I remember having heard faintly the beautiful piano music of Mozart and Bach. Subsequently, after the operation, I was almost a little sad that these unique moments had come to an end. The post-operative medical care was very meticulous, in a warm, serene atmosphere in which one feels cared for.

I was so happy with my "new face" that I went to a professional photographer to have some pictures done. My daughter, who at that time had suggested I undergo the face lift, subsequently turned out to be almost a bit jealous when young men looked at me. My husband, my friends and colleagues all thought that the effect of rejuvenation was fantastic and so natural. A surgical rejuvenation of the face is first and foremost a personal move, which you do for yourself. My operation aroused a great deal of curiosity, especially from my nephew, who's a doctor. He couldn't believe that I felt absolutely no pain and recovered so quickly and that I could take up my sporting activities after a week already. I can recommend a face lift to all those who feel they need it. They should not hesitate one single moment.

Mrs. Gisèle Decheverens, Geneva

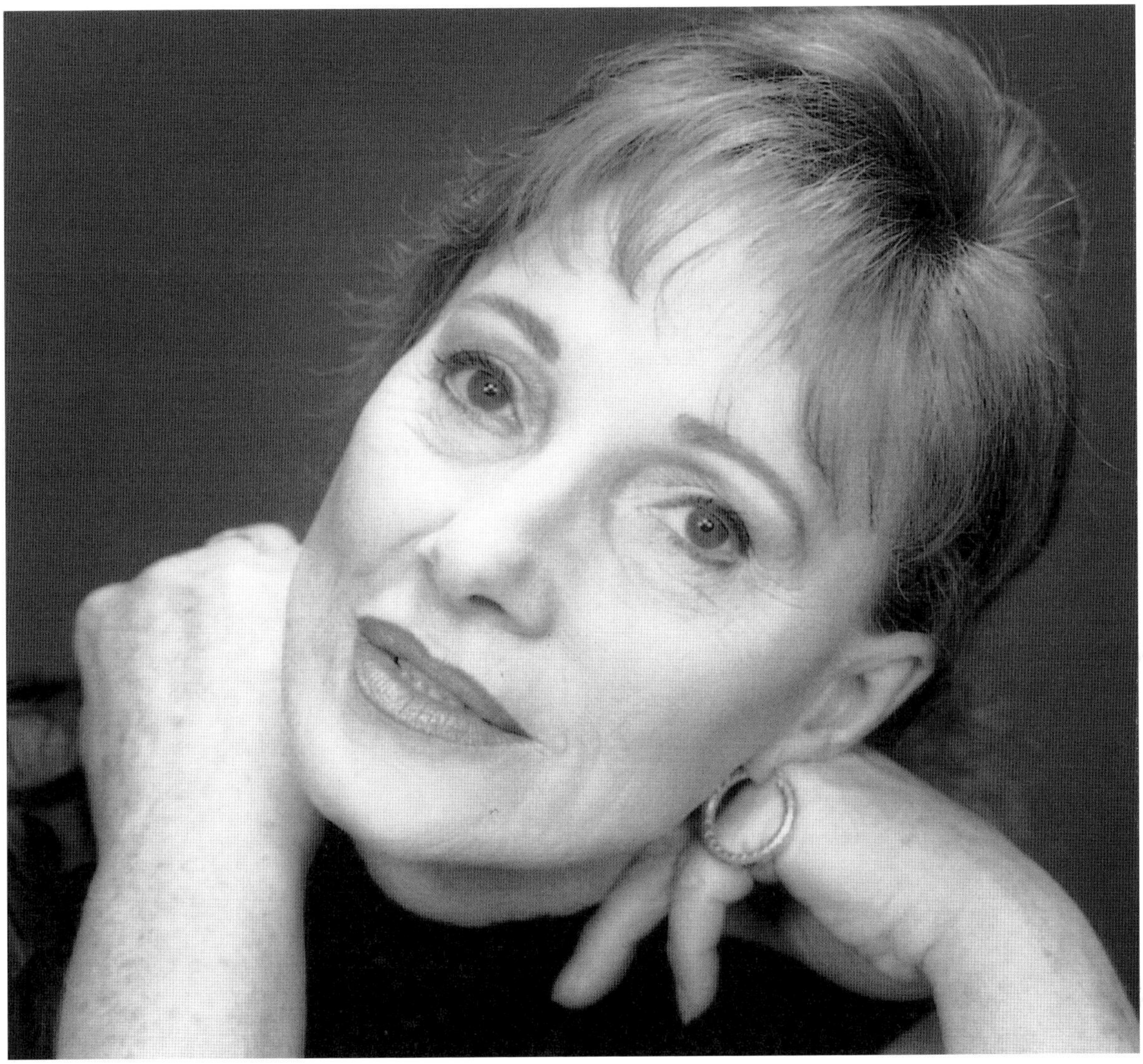

Gisèle Dechevrens

Photographic credits

The publisher, Benteli Verlag, and Urs Victor Burki wish to thank the museums and photographers for the reproduction rights they have granted. We have made every effort to identify copyright holders of the illustrations. However, if we have failed to inform anyone, we ask them to contact the publisher.

Agence photographique Roger-Viollet, Paris: fig. 7, p. 14

Archaeological Museum, Olympia: fig. 4, p. 33

Archiv für Kunst und Geschichte, akg-images, Berlin: fig. 18, p. 31

Biblioteca Ambrosiana, Milano: fig. 22, p. 42

Biblioteca Reale di Torino, su concessione del Ministero per i Beni e le Attività Culturali: fig. 8, p. 36; fig. 11, p. 37

Bildarchiv Preussischer Kulturbesitz, Berlin: fig. 1, p. 21

British Museum, London, The Trustees of the British Museum: fig. 2, p. 12; fig. 2, p. 27

Egyptian Museum, Cairo: fig. 3, p. 23

Fondazione Casa Buonarroti, Firenze: fig. 23, p. 43

Galleria dell'Accademia, Campo della Carità, Venezia: fig. 9, p. 36; fig. 10, p. 36

Galleria Nazionale delle Marche, Urbino, su concessione del Ministero per i Beni e le Attività Culturali, Soprintendenza per il Patrimonio delle Marche, Urbino: fig. 4, p. 12

Hirmer Verlag GmbH, München, aus Kurt Lange und Max Hirmer, Ägypten: Architektur, Plastik, Malerei in drei Jahrtausenden, München, Hirmer 1967: fig. 2, p. 22

Musée du Louvre, Paris, photo RMN / Hervé Lewandowski / Thierry Le Mage: fig. 6, p.13

Musée du Louvre, Paris, photo RMN / Hervé Lewandowski: fig. 8, p. 25; fig. 1, p. 32; fig. 2, p. 33; fig. 28, p. 47

Musée du Louvre, Paris, photo RMN / Michèle Bellot: fig. 3, p.12

Musée du Louvre, Paris, photo RMN / Daniel Arnaudet: fig. 15, p. 39

Musée du Louvre, Paris, photo RMN / Harry Bréjat: fig. 18, p. 41

Musée du Louvre, Paris, photo RMN / Christian Jean: fig. 19, p. 41

Museo Archeologico Nazionale, Napoli, su concessione del Ministero per i Beni e le Attività Culturali: fig. 4, p. 24; fig. 1, p. 26

Museo e Gallerie Nazionali di Capodimonte, Napoli: fig. 12, p. 36

Museo Nazionale di Taranto, su concessione del Ministero per i Beni e le Attività Culturali, Soprintendenza per i Beni Archeologici della Puglia: fig. 5, p. 34

Muzeum Narodowym w Krakowie, Fondation K. Czartoryski, Krakau: fig. 21, p. 42

National Archaeological Museum, Athens: fig. 3, S. 33; fig. 3, p. 27; fig. 4, p. 27

Orell Füssli Verlag AG, Zürich, aus: István Rácz: Antikes Erbe, Meisterwerke aus Schweizer Sammlungen, Zürich: Orell Füssli 1965, p. 120: fig. 6, p. 25; p. 142: fig. 7, p. 25

Polo Museale Fiorentino, Galleria degli Uffizi, su concessione del Ministero per i Beni e le Attività Culturali, Firenze: fig. 7, p. 35; fig. 17, p. 40

Polo Museale Fiorentino, Museo Nazionale del Bargello, su concessione del Ministero per i Beni e le Attività Culturali, Firenze: fig. 6a, p. 34, fig. 6b, p. 35

Polo Museale Fiorentino, Galleria Palatina, su concessione del Ministero per i Beni e le Attività Culturali, Firenze: fig. 5, p.12

The Picture Desk, London: fig. 5, p. 24

The Pierpont Morgan Library, New York, Department of photographic services, rights and reproductions: fig. 13b, p. 39